History of Stroke

History of Stroke

Editors

Julien Bogousslavsky
Maurizio Paciaroni
Michael G. Hennerici
Laurent Tatu

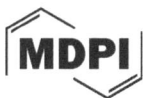

Basel • Beijing • Wuhan • Barcelona • Belgrade • Novi Sad • Cluj • Manchester

Editors
Julien Bogousslavsky
Center for Brain and Nervous System Diseases
Swiss Medical Network, Clinique Valmont
Glion, Switzerland

Maurizio Paciaroni
Santa Maria della Misericordia Hospital,
University of Perugia
Perugia (Italy)

Michael G. Hennerici
University of Heidelberg
Mannheim/Heidelberg, Germany

Laurent Tatu
CHU Besançon - University of Franche-Comté
Besançon, France

Editorial Office
MDPI
St. Alban-Anlage 66
4052 Basel, Switzerland

For citation purposes, cite each chapter independently as indicated below:

Lastname, Firstname, Firstname Lastname, and Firstname Lastname. Year. Chapter Title. In *Book Title*. Edited by Editor 1 and Editor 2. Series Title (optional). Basel: MDPI, Page Range.

ISBN 978-3-0365-2314-9 (Hbk)
ISBN 978-3-0365-2313-2 (PDF)
doi.org/10.3390/books978-3-0365-2313-2

© 2023 by the authors. Articles in this book are Open Access and distributed under the Creative Commons Attribution (CC BY) license. The book as a whole is distributed by MDPI under the terms and conditions of the Creative Commons Attribution-NonCommercial-NoDerivs (CC BY-NC-ND) license.

Contents

About the Editors vii

Preface ix

Contributors xi

Part I: Encephalic Arteries, 'Apolplexy' and 'Brain Softening'

1) The Discovery of Encephalic Arteries—A Historical Overview 2
2) The Evolving Concepts of Apoplexy and Brain Softening 18
3) Introduction to the Terms Arteriosclerosis, Thrombosis and Embolism 27
4) The Turning Point in Stroke Investigation for Neurologists 30
5) Stroke and the Arts 37

Part II: The 20th Century Revolution

6) The Interest in the Pathology and Pathophysiology of Vascular Lesions 54
7) History of Cardiac Embolism 68
8) History of "Lacunar Infarction" 73
9) History of Vascular Cognitive Impairment and Dementia 80

Part III: Progress in Diagnosis and Treatment: The Last 50 Years

10) Progress in Diagnosis and Treatment: The Last 50 Years of Stroke Prevention 91
11) History of Stroke Imaging 102
12) Stroke Units, Stroke Registries and Acute Management (R)evolutions 113
13) From Thrombolysis, to Thrombectomy in Acute Ischemic Stroke 120
14) The History of Clinical Neuroprotection Failure 130
15) Stroke Rehabilitation from a Historical Perspective 139

About the Editors

Julien Bogousslavsky, a former full professor of neurology and head of university department of neurology in Switzerland, now chairs the Center for brain and nervous system disorders of the Swiss Medical Network, along with his position of Chief editor of European Neurology, the third oldest neurological journal. He was founder of the European Stroke Conference and of the journal Cerebrovascular Diseases along with Michael Hennerici, and was the millenium president of the International Stroke Society. He has published over 700 scientific papers and books, and is also the author of works and brain and creativity, writers such as Marcel Proust or Blaise Cendrars, Surrealism, and the relationships between avant-garde poets and artists.

Maurizio Paciaroni, having completed his 4-year university specialization course in Neurology, at the University of Perugia in Italy, went on to became a Research Fellow in the field of vascular neurology at the University of Lausanne in Switzerland. Subsequently, he participated in NASCET (North American Symptomatic Carotid Endarterectomy Trial) at the Robarts Research Institute, the University of Western Ontario, London Ontario, Canada. Currently, he is the team leader of the Stroke Unit at the University of Perugia Hospital, Italy. He has published more than 250 research papers, in both English and Italian, and has co-authored several chapters and texts on stroke.

Michael G. Hennerici is professor emeritus and former chairman of the department of neurology as well as medical director of the Mannheim Hospital at the University of Heidelberg, Germany. Along with Julien Bogousslavsky (Switzerland) he was founder and chairman of the European Stroke Conference (ESC) in 1990 (Düsseldorf, Germany) and the journal Cerebrovascular Diseases (Honorary Editor and Founding Editor in Chief) for more than a quarter of a century. He has published more than 850 scientific papers and books on all aspects of research in basic neurophysiology as well as imaging principles of the brain and its vasculature (Ultrasound, CT and MRI), all aspects of Cerebrovascular Diseases (eg. diagnosis, management and treatment in exploratory pilot and large clinical trials) and pioneer studies of the Natural History of Asymptomatic Carotid Disease in particular (1987). Along with his wife Marion Hennerici, who early joined the ESC Executive Committee, he founded the European Stroke Research Foundation (ESRF), which today continuously supports numerous applications of researchers worldwide (https://www.esrf.website). Following his primary education in musical arts (Organist diploma) and numerous concerts given, he later became interested in brain diseases of musicians and painting artists as well as their relationships to stroke.This also follows the spirits of education at the Department of Neurology and Neurophysiology in Freiburg im Breisgau, Germany during his student's education in the early 1970s.

Laurent Tatu is professor of anatomy and neurologist. He is the coordinator of the Department of Anatomy at the University of Franche-Comté (France) and head of the Neuromuscular Diseases Department at Besançon University Hospital. His main research topics are vascular anatomy of the brain and morphological and functional muscle anatomy applied to botulinum toxin therapy for neurological diseases. He is an associate editor of the journals "European Neurology" and "Case Reports in Neurology". With a longstanding interest in history, he is the author of works on the history of medicine and the history of the First World War. With Julien Bogousslavsky, he has published numerous articles on the history of medicine and three books on neuropsychiatry in the First World War (2012), Blaise Cendrars (2015) and Gustave Roussy (2023).

Preface

It is fashionable today to say that one wants to live in the present moment. But beyond this simple cliché, one forgets what "the present" corresponds to. Indeed, to be somewhat provocative, the present is never really present, since it immediately disappears to be replaced by another momentum, which also disappears, and so on. The future also does not exist. So, what does exist or is at least more stable when one considers the passage of time? The past. In fact, the past, i.e., "history", is what precisely defines what we are today, how we experience the transience of the "here and now", and how we may plan what is coming next. For this reason, like in all human sciences, history is of utmost importance to understand events, developments, successes, and failures in medicine. In addition, at the neurophysiological level, this corresponds well to the general functioning of the brain, which is based on acquired patterns, i.e., "memory" in the broadest sense. Thus, one could say that the appropriate integration of the past is the sine qua non condition for a normal present life and future planning.

Given the importance of the brain and nervous system in general in human activities, the history of neurology and neuroscience is a truly privileged and particularly fascinating field in the history of medicine. In this domain, however, very little has been written on the historical evolution of cerebrovascular disease and stroke. This may be due to the fact that stroke has often been classified in the border zone—sometimes a no man's land—between internal medicine, angiology, and neurology. For instance, when I started my training, practicing and academic neurologists seemed much more interested in diseases of the nerves and muscles than stroke. In many countries, brain lesion management was left to neurosurgeons. And I remember the smiles and laughs of more senior colleagues when my chief appointed me as a consultant to the "division of hemiplegia", which at the time belonged to internal medicine in the hospital. As is often the case, however, the punishment could be transformed into a positive experience. Indeed, beyond the therapeutic issues, which at the time were rather limited, I discovered that strokes were probably the easiest, most common, and most interesting way to understand how focal brain lesions may affect neurological function, including changes in complex phenomena, such as behavior. Along with therapeutic progress, stroke subsequently acquired better interest from clinicians in general, and it has now become a very significant field of academic and clinical neurology.

While its particular historical development may have inhibited extensive research on its evolution over the centuries, it is also the reason why this topic is of particular interest today, with large parts still waiting to be studied. To my knowledge, the first attempt to publish a book on the history of stroke was by William Fields and Noreen Lemak in 1989. However, it placed a strong emphasis on ancient texts, which made it not so easy to read by non-scholars, given the dramatic changes in medicine from antiquity to modern times. This is why we have decided to focus the present book on more recent history, mainly from the nineteenth century up to the most recent advances in stroke diagnosis and management, when this picture can give a striking impression of the fascinating chronological developments in the stroke field over the last two hundred years. This is also the process we followed after we launched the European Stroke Conference in 1990 with Michael Hennerici in introducing historical overviews in the scientific program as often as possible.

In the following chapters, the concepts of apoplexy and brain softening, atheroma–thrombosis–embolism, and small versus large artery disease have been traced over the decades, with a focus on investigations, diagnosis, and treatment, including prevention, acute therapy, and rehabilitation. Because of their specific interest associated with historical issues, some other topics have also been covered, such as vascular cognitive impairment or the influence of stroke on art.

Along with my co-editors, I am deeply grateful to the authors of the following chapters who have provided thorough, innovative, and stimulating overviews of these topics from a historical perspective. One of the goals of this book is to trigger interest in the history of neurology in general through the periscope of the history of cerebrovascular disease and stroke. Indeed, probably even more than in other domains, the field of stroke history has been only partially explored, and many fascinating topics in this field remain to be studied.

Julien Bogousslavsky **for the Editors** *Maurizio Paciaroni, Michael G. Hennerici*
and *Laurent Tatu*
Editors

Contributors

Bartlomiej Piechowski-Jozwiak
Staff Physician
Neurological Institute, Cleveland Clinic Abu Dhabi, The United Arab Emirates; Honorary Consultant Neurologist
King's College Hospital, Denmark Hill, London, UK

Carmen Calvello
Neurology Unit, Department of Systems Medicine, University of Rome Tor Vergata, Rome, Italy

Frederic Assal
Médecin Hôpitaux Universitaires de Genève et Faculté de médecine

Giacomo Baso
"Luigi Sacco" Department of Biomedical and Clinical Sciences, University of Milan

Giorgio Silvestrelli
Stroke Unit, Department of Neuroscience
ASST Mantova, Italy

Giacomo Staffolani
Stroke Unit and Division of Cardiovascular Medicine, University of Perugia, Italy

Jukka Putaala
Neurology, Helsinki University Hospital and University of Helsinki, Helsinki, Finland

Julien Bogousslavsky
Clinique Valmont Route de Valmont 1823 Glion sur Montreux

Kateryna Antonenko
Department of Neurology, Inselspital, University Hospital and University of Bern, Bern, 3010, Switzerland

Laurent Tatu
Department of Neuromuscular diseases and Department of Anatomy. CHU Besançon - University of Franche-Comté Besançon, France

Leonardo Pantoni
"Luigi Sacco" Department of Biomedical and Clinical Sciences, University of Milan

Lucia Gentili
Department of Neurology and Stroke Unit, USL Umbria1, Città di Castello, Italy

Lukas Sveikata
Chef de Clinique scientifique
Hôpitaux Universitaires de Genève et Faculté de médecine

Maria Giulia Mosconi
Clinical Researcher Santa Maria Della Misericordia Hospital-University of Perugia, Cardiovascular Medicine-Stroke Unit, Perugia, Italy

Maurizio Paciaroni
Stroke Unit and Division of Cardiovascular Medicine, University of Perugia, Italy

Mauro Zampolini
Neurologia-Stroke Unit, Dipartimento di Neuroriabilitazione, Ospedale S. Giovanni Battista, USLUmbria 2

Michael G. Hennerici
University of Heidelberg, Heidelberg, Germany

Michela Giustozzi
Stroke Unit and Division of Cardiovascular Medicine, University of Perugia, Italy

Monica Acciarresi
Neurologia-Stroke Unit, Dipartimento di Neuroriabilitazione, Ospedale S. Giovanni Battista, USLUmbria 2

Norbert Nighoghossian
University Claude Bernard Lyon

Olivier Walusinski
Family Physician, Private practice Lauréat de l'Académie de Médecine (Paris)

Roberta Rinaldi
Department of Neurology and Stroke Unit, San Giovanni Battista Hospital, Foligno, 06034, Italy

Stephen Meairs
University of Heidelberg, Heidelberg, Germany

Part I: Encephalic Arteries, 'Apolplexy' and 'Brain Softening'

The Discovery of Encephalic Arteries—A Historical Overview

Laurent Tatu and Julien Bogousslavsky

Abstract: The knowledge of the anatomy of brain arteries developed in two main phases. The first, mainly descriptive, was the discovery of the main arteries at the base of the brain. The second was the study of the branching patterns of these arteries using more specific anatomical techniques, such as intra-arterial injection. The great anatomo-clinical work of Charles Foix (1882–1927), the first true stroke neurologist, enabled the transformation of these anatomical data into a form directly applicable to clinical practice.

1. Introduction

The names of some vessels, such as the vein of Galen and the torcular Herophili, suggest that our understanding of cerebral vascular anatomy dates back to Antiquity, but this is not, in fact, the case: for many centuries, anatomical representations of the brain completely omitted the blood vessels. Knowledge of vascular anatomy came much later, and, as in other medical specialties, did not immediately lead to any improvement in patient care.

Parenchymal cerebral anatomy and vascular anatomy were ultimately brought together by pathology. The discovery of arterial lesions (arteriosclerosis, arterial embolisms, etc.) and their role in cerebral lesions (apoplexy, softening, etc.) provided the link between the arteries and the brain.

In this chapter, we highlight the key milestones in the understanding of the cerebral circulation before the advent of neuro-imagery, from the discovery of these arteries to modern anatomo-clinical research. Many anatomical errors, both ancient, such as the concept of a human rete mirabile, and more recent, such as l'artère de la fossette latérale du bulbe (artery of the lateral medullary fossa), have hindered our understanding of the blood supply to the brain.

The knowledge of brain vessel anatomy developed in two main phases. The first, mainly descriptive, was the discovery of the main arteries at the base of the brain. The second was the study of the branching patterns of these arteries using more specific anatomical techniques, such as intra-arterial injection. The great anatomo-clinical work of Charles Foix (1882–1927), the first true stroke neurologist, enabled the transformation of these anatomical data into a form directly applicable to clinical practice.

2. The First Mentions of the Cerebral Vessels

In ancient Greece, anatomy was not a major part of medical education, which was greatly influenced by Hippocrates' humoral theory. Additionally, the Greeks considered dead bodies to be sacred, which meant that there were very few dissections of human cadavers. Some animal dissections and possibly fetal dissections were performed, but there was little interest in the brain, which was considered secondary to the heart.

In the third century BCE, the Hellenistic Alexandria established by the Ptolemaic Pharaohs became a renowned seat of learning for many well-known Greek physicians. Over a period of around fifty years, some of these physicians, particularly Herophilus of Chalcedon (ca 330–ca 250 BCE) and Erasistratus of Chios (ca 315–ca 240 BCE), dissected human cadavers. Herophilus specialized in brain anatomy. Fragments of his treatises have survived in the writings of more recent anatomists, although they have been translated multiple times in the interim [1,2]. Herophilus seems to have distinguished between arteries and veins, but his interest in the brain focused mainly on cerebral ventricles, meninges, and superficial veins. Notably, he discovered and named the confluence of dural sinuses near the internal occipital protuberance, a confluence that later bore his name—the torcular Herophili [1].

In the second century CE, the anatomical contributions of Galen (ca 129–ca 210) based on animal dissections established him as an influential figure. Galen was born in a Greek family in the city of Pergamum in Asia Minor. He undertook part of his medical training in Alexandria and subsequently moved to Rome, where he lived for most of his life. He had likely never dissected human cadavers, but his anatomical and physiological ideas based on animal models were regarded as immutable by the medieval world for centuries [3].

Galen developed the fictional concept of rete mirabile, which gained an impressive influence in the history of brain anatomy. The rete mirabile is an elaborate network of fine vessels into which the carotid arteries divide at the base of the brain. It exists only in ungulates, not in the human brain. The fragments of text attributed to the Alexandrian school of anatomy credit Herophilus of Chalcedoine with what appears to be the first description of the rete mirabile in an animal [1].

Galen transposed the rete mirabile from dissections of the ox onto the human brain [4]. The rete mirabile played a central role in the Galenic concept of physiology, which was also based on other fictional ideas. For example, food absorbed by the gut underwent "concoction" and then was transported by the blood to the liver, where it was imbued with "natural spirit". The blood then left the liver and travelled via the veins to the right ventricle of the heart, where impurities were exhaled through the lungs. It then entered the left ventricle through the pores of the inter-ventricular septum. There, the blood was imbued with a higher form of pneuma: the "vital spirits" drawn from the outside by inhalation through the lungs. This blood, along with its associated "natural spirits", travelled via the arteries to the brain and entered the rete mirabile at the base of the brain, where the blood was charged with the final and highest form of pneuma, the "animal spirits". The ventricles of the brain were the final repository of the "animal spirits", which flowed out of the brain through the nerves to the organs of the body. According to Galen, the convolutions of the rete mirabile were necessary for slowing the passage of blood, allowing the transformation of natural spirits into animal spirits [5].

The medieval times were deeply influenced by this Galenic vision and the ventricular conception of brain function, which also had a significant impact on Arabic medicine. During this period, Mondino dei Luzzi (ca 1275–1326), professor at the University of Bologna, was one of the first anatomists to have reintroduced the dissection of human cadavers to anatomy teaching. One section of his book Anathomia, written in around 1316, deals with the anatomy of the skull, brain, eyes, and ears. The description is focused on the medieval theory of the brain as cerebral chambers, without clear insight into the question of the cerebral arteries. Mondino also perpetuated the Galenic vision of the brain. The first illustrated version of Mondino's work was created by Guido da Vigevano (ca 1280–ca 1349) [6].

A rare medieval representation of the brain that dates from the mid-13th century and whose illustrator is unknown includes some cerebral and vertebral vessels and probably the rete mirabile [7] (Figure 1A). Other medieval anatomical depictions of the brain were still based on the ventricular and rete mirabile concepts. The depiction in 1501 of a human head in Antropologium de hominis dignitate (1501) by Magnus Hundt (1449–1519) of the University of Leipzig is a clear example of this [8] (Figure 1B).

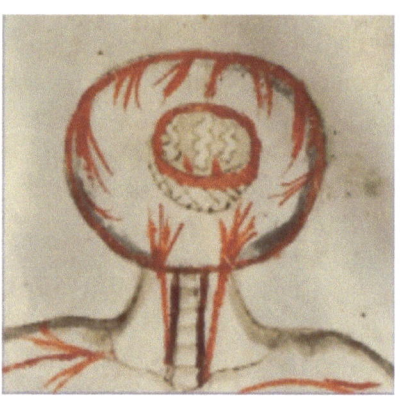
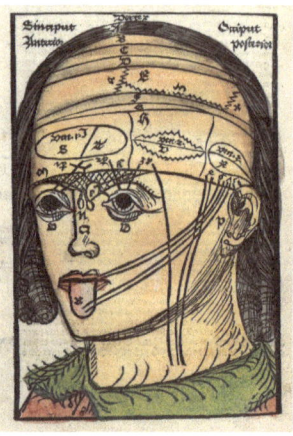

A
B

Figure 1. (**A**) Medieval representation of the brain including some cerebral and vertebral vessels and probably the rete mirabile (mid-13th century). Reprinted from [7], used with permission. (**B**) Depiction of a human head (1501) by Magnus Hundt (1449–1519). Reprinted from [8], used with permission.

3. The Slow Transition from the Rete Mirabile to the Cerebral Arterial Circle

The end of the 15th century marked the beginning of a new era for brain anatomy, an era that frequently challenged Galen's ideas. Initially rooted in the Italian universities, this resurgence of anatomy progressively involved scholars from across Europe and culminated with the major anatomical work of Andreas Vesalius (1514–1564). One of the debates was the existence of the rete mirabile in humans, which had rarely been questioned before then.

Among the pre-Vesalian anatomists, the Italian physician Jacobus Berengarius Carpensis (Berengario da Carpi) (ca 1460–ca 1530), a professor at the University of Bologna who introduced anatomical illustrations based on nature, was one of the first to deny the presence of the rete mirabile in humans. In his Commentaria on Mondino's Anathomia (1521) and Isagogae breves (1523), he reported that he had dissected around 100 heads but had failed to discover a rete mirabile [9,10].

The Flemish-born anatomist and physician Andreas Vesalius (Andries Wytinck van Wesel) re-established anatomy as an observational science after a long period of stagnation under the teachings of Galen. He was appointed as a professor of surgery and anatomy at Padua University, where he dissected human cadavers and relied heavily on anatomical drawings to support his teaching. In 1538, Vesalius published the Tabulae Anatomicae Sex, which included an illustration of the rete mirabile that he called "mirabilis plexus reticularis" (wonderful plexus network) [11]. At first, Vesalius still believed in the existence of a rete mirabile in humans, but comparative dissections of human and animal cadavers ultimately convinced him that Galen must have been wrong.

In 1543, Vesalius published his magnum opus, De humani corporis fabrica. Liber VII of the Fabrica, which includes a systematic dissection of the brain, illustrated with woodcut prints through 12 sequential stages. He now denied the existence of the rete mirabile in humans and castigated himself for his prior failure to recognize this error [12]. Nevertheless, the idea of the rete mirabile in humans did not disappear after Vesalius but remained part of the medico-anatomical discourse [13]. The discovery of the brain circulation by William Harvey (1578–1657) only had a small impact on the understanding of the cerebral arteries and the discussion around the rete mirabile.

From the Renaissance, the concept of the rete mirabile slowly evolved into the concept of the major anastomotic arterial system, which became one of the most famous eponymous structures of the human body: the circle of Willis. Thomas Willis (1621–1675), a physician at Oxford, demonstrated this anastomotic arterial structure with great precision, which is in fact an arterial heptagon [14].

Before Willis' accurate description and illustration, some other anatomists had evoked such a structure [15]. Gabriele Fallopius (Fallopio) (1523–1562), professor of anatomy at Padua University, described the arterial circle in Observationes anatomicae (1561), but his description was incomplete and he underestimated this anastomotic system [16]. An anatomical plate from Tabulae anatomicae by Giulio Casserio (Casserius) (1545–1605) provided an incomplete illustration of the arteries of the basal brain that also included a rete mirabile branching out from the carotid artery. Casserius' Tabulae anatomicae were incorporated into De humani corporis fabrica (1627) by Adrianus Spigelius (van der Spieghel) (1567–1625) after the death of both anatomists [17]. The German anatomist Johann Vesling (Veslingus, Wesling) (1595–1649), also a professor of anatomy in Padua, provided, in his second edition of the Syntagma (1647), an incomplete description and illustration of the anastomotic arteries. In his description, some branches that did not come from the carotid artery and that spread out on the basal face of the brain corresponded to the presumed rete mirabile [18] (Figure 2A).

Johann Jakob Wepfer (1620–1695), a Swiss physician from Schaffhausen, is usually regarded as the true discoverer of the arterial circle. Six years before Willis' publication, Wepfer published his Observationes anatomicae ex cadaveribus eorum, quos sustulit apoplexia cum exercitatione de ejus loco affecto (1658) [19]. In this work, Wepfer clearly described this anastomotic system, demonstrating that he knew the arterial organization of the base of the brain in detail. Unfortunately, he did not provide an illustration of the arterial circle but referred to one in Vestling's Syntagma.

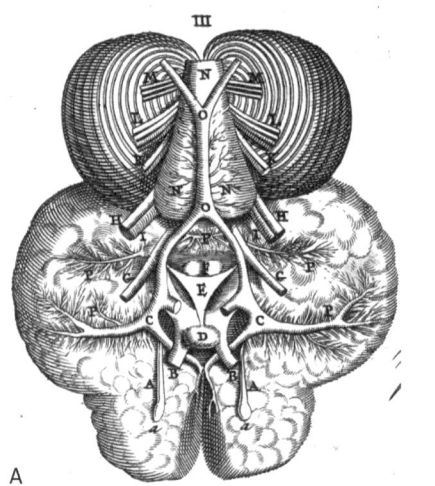 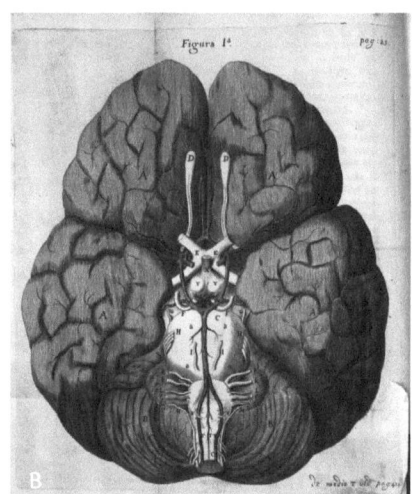

Figure 2. (**A**) Representation of the arteries of the base of the brain by Johann Vesling (1595–1649). Some arterial branches (P) correspond to the presumed rete mirabile. Reprinted from [18], used with permission. (**B**) First illustration of the arterial circle of the base of the brain in 1664 by Thomas Willis (1621–1675) Reprinted from [14], used with permission.

Thomas Willis—assisted by Richard Lower (1631–1691) and the architect Christopher Wren (1632–1723), who provided the drawings—added little new information to Wepfer's description, despite using new dissection techniques on human cadavers. However, he gave the first complete illustration of the circle in both man and sheep in 1664 (Figure 2B). The pictorial representations of these share certain inaccuracies, but his illustration highlighting the relationships between nerves and vessels is superior to those of his predecessors. As a physician, Willis also tried to understand the functional role of the anastomotic system [14].

Throughout the following century, the question of the existence of the rete mirabile in man continued to parasitize the anatomical perspective of the basal brain [20]. The French anatomist Raymond de Vieussens (ca 1541–1715) in his Neurographia universalis (1684) and the English physician Humphrey Ridley (1653–1708) in his Anatomy of the brain (1695), among others, continued to defend the idea of the existence of a rete mirabile in humans, despite knowledge of the circle [21,22]. The idea was more firmly ruled out from the mid-18th century.

4. The Time of Injection Studies

At the end of 18th century, Félix Vicq d'Azyr (1748–1794) elegantly illustrated the arteries of the base of the brain [23] (Figure 3). Nevertheless, brain and artery anatomy were still considered independently, as reflected in Samuel Thomas Soemmering's (1755–1830) anatomical book Vom Baue des menschlichen Körpers, which treated the angiology and anatomy of the brain in two separate volumes [24]. In the first quarter of the 19th century, brain anatomy was still focused on parenchymal anatomy, with numerous controversies concerning the craniology and phrenology described by Franz-Joseph Gall (1758–1828) and Johann Gaspar Spurzheim (1776–1832).

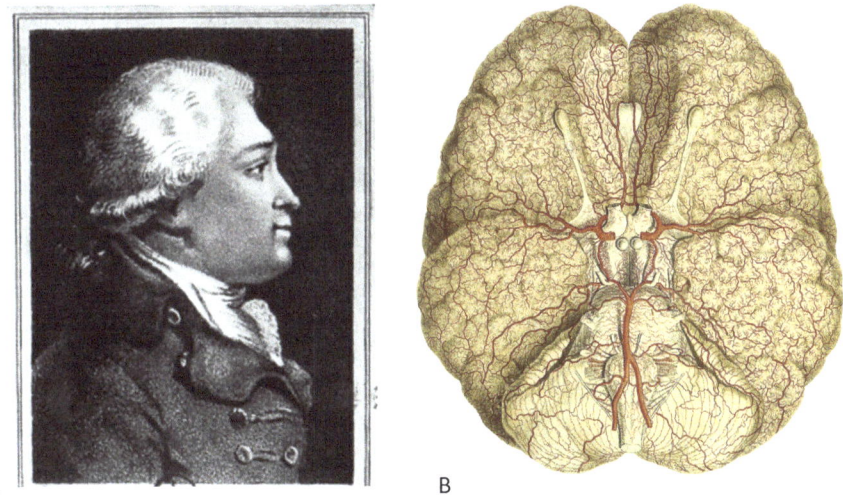

Figure 3. (**A**) Félix Vicq d'Azyr (1748–1794) (Public domain). (**B**) Illustration of the arteries of the base of the brain by Vicq d'Azyr. Reprinted from [23], used with permission.

Although slow, the emergence of arterial pathological concepts eventually brought to light the close relationships between arterial abnormalities and brain lesions. The seminal works of Jean André Rochoux (1787–1852) and Léon Rostan (1790–1866) introduced the concept of brain softening as an entity distinct from apoplexy, which is now regarded as a hemorrhagic phenomenon [25,26]. In 1829, Jean-Frédéric Lobstein (1777–1835) used the term "arteriosclerosis" to define abnormal deposits on the arterial wall [27]. A few years later, the German pathologist Rudolf Virchow (1821–1902) clarified the terms "thrombosis" and "embolism", and coined the term "ischemia" to describe the consequences of a lack of arterial flow to an organ [28].

In this new pathological context, some anatomists decided to study the branching patterns of the main cerebral arteries coming from the arterial circle at the base of the brain or from the vertebro-basilar system. They used more sophisticated anatomical procedures, such as intra-arterial injections using syringes and liquor dyed with ink, a technique that had been used by Thomas Willis and the Oxford group two centuries earlier.

In 1872, the German physician Otto Heubner (1843–1926) was likely the first to investigate the distribution of the branches of the cerebral arteries, in an injection study performed on 30 brains. He injected each artery with a colored liquor and noted the structures supplied. He defined the cortical and central territories of brain arteries and demonstrated that the posterior communicating artery supplies the anterior part of thalamus and the anterior choroidal artery supplies the posterior limb of the internal capsule. He also described a small artery arising close to the anterior communicating artery that provides blood to the head of the corpus striatum. This artery was later named the recurrent branch of anterior cerebral artery but nowadays bears his name: the recurrent artery of Heuber [29].

Henri Duret (1849–1921), a pupil of Jean-Martin Charcot and later a professor of surgery in Lille, also conducted impressive anatomical work [30]. In 1873–1874, Duret, using an injection technique that he did not record and an unspecified number of brains, classified encephalic arteries using a morphogenetic approach. He also published diagrams describing the different distributions of the anterior, middle, and posterior cerebral arteries [31,32] (Figure 4A). He presented the first study on the distribution of the arteries supplying the medulla oblongata [33].

Duret also focused on the arterial vascularization of the deep grey nuclei of the brain, introducing the concept of the lenticulo-optic arteries (pédicule lenticulo-optique) whose existence would be highly debated in the following years [31]. Jean Martin Charcot (1825–1893), the great French neurologist, had little interest in stroke [34], but he nevertheless defended and diffused the work of Duret in his published Leçons. He presented the lenticulo-optic arteries and emphasized the role of another lenticulo-striate artery mainly involved in brain hemorrhage, later sometimes called Charcot's artery [35] (Figure 4B).

In 1891, the Austrian anatomist Alexander Kolisko (1857–1918) performed an injection study of the anterior choroidal artery in 17 brains. He described both its cortical and deep territories and confirmed Heubner's results concerning its involvement in the vascularization of the posterior limb of the internal capsule [36].

The years 1907–1910 were very fruitful for the understanding of brain vascularization. In 1907, the Boston physician James Bourne Ayer (1882–1963) and Hamlet Frederick Aitken (1872–1939), artist at the Massachusetts hospital, published a first detailed report on the arteries of the corpus striatum. They confirmed Heubner's views on the participation of the anterior cerebral artery in the corpus striatum supply [37]. A few months later, Hamlet Frederick Aitken made drawings from fresh dissections of numerous brains and confirmed the participation of the anterior choroidal artery in the vascularization of the corpus striatum. They denied the existence of the so-called Charcot's artery and Duret's lenticulo-optic arteries [38]. Duret replied to Aitken in a paper published in 1910 and accepted the development of some new arterial concepts but maintained his view on the anterior cerebral artery and lenticulo-optic arteries [39].

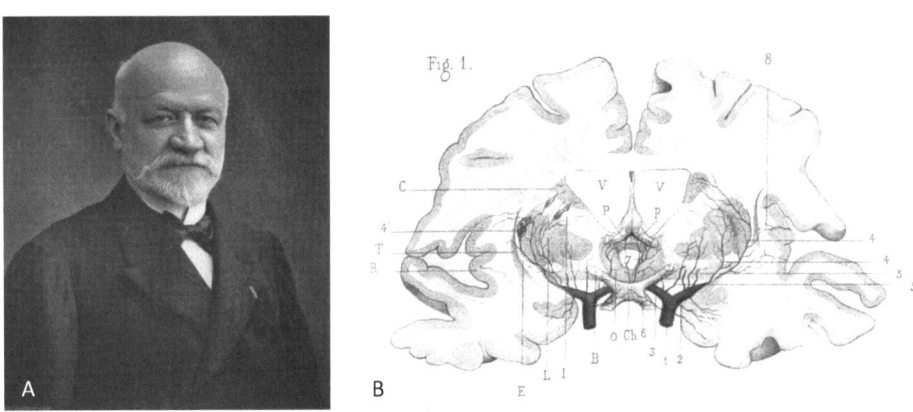

Figure 4. (**A**) Henri Duret (1849–1921) (Public domain). (**B**) Frontal section of the brain from Duret's work showing the lenticulo-striate arteries including Charcot's artery (4). Reprinted from [31], used with permission.

In the same period, the British anatomist Charles Edward Beevor (1854–1908) presented the results of seven years of arterial brain injection studies [40] (Figure 5A). Beevor injected nearly 100 brains using a different technique to that used by Duret and Heubner. Beevor used colored gelatin to inject the main brain arteries individually, including the posterior communicating and anterior choroidal arteries, following a strict and ingenious methodology [41]. His detailed results were presented in an attractive and colorful way. Beevor published the first type of brain mapping, displaying both the anatomical structures and the arterial territories in horizontal, frontal and sagittal brain sections [42] (Figure 5B).

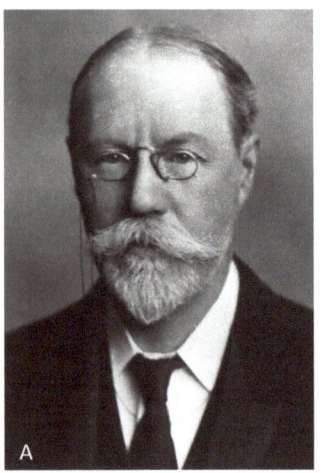 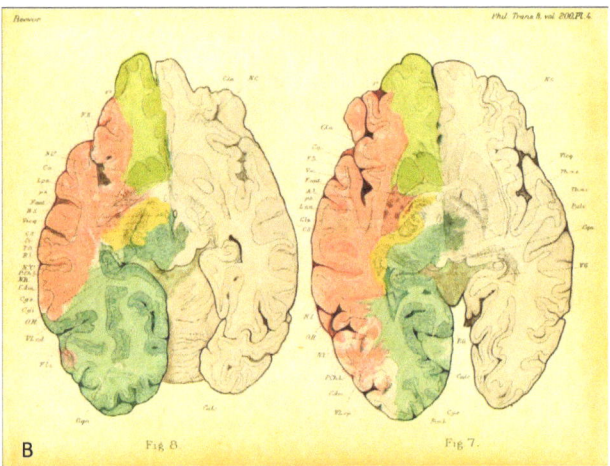

Figure 5. (**A**) Charles E. Beevor (1854–1908) (Public domain). (**B**) Horizontal brain section from Beevor's arterial brain mapping. Reprinted from [42], used with permission.

Initial works using arterial injection raised the question of the variability of the cortical artery territories and the existence of anastomoses. In his initial papers and in his 1910 article, Duret stated that there was little to no variation and that the anastomoses between the territories were too small to be of significance [31,39]. Beevor was the first to suggest a clear variability in the cortical territories of the main cerebral arteries [41].

5. Charles Foix and the Modern Era of Neurovascular Anatomy

Charles Foix (1882–1927) began his career at the Paris school of clinical anatomy, where he was a student of Pierre Marie (1853–1940). His career was interrupted by World War One, which he spent on the front in the Balkans. After qualifying as a doctor after the war, he became a professor at the Paris medical school in 1923, and he took the post of Head of Department at the Hospice des incurables d'Ivry the following year. Foix was an accomplished poet and lyricist. His death in 1927 from a perforated gastric ulcer prematurely ended his career [43] (Figure 6A).

From 1923 to 1927, Foix focused his research on the cerebral blood supply, using anatomical injection techniques—sometimes paired with the use of X-rays—anatomo-pathological studies, and anatomo-clinical correlations. He re-examined Duret's work, which was by this time somewhat outdated and of little practical use. Foix published multiple articles that became the foundations of a new discipline, of which he was the first true proponent—vascular neurology. His work was performed with the help of his interns, notably his primary collaborator, Pierre Hillemand (1895–1979).

Charles Foix made rapid progress, but these advancements occured in stages. The first step was the individualization of the vascular territory of the posterior cerebral artery [44]. Foix and Hillemand then defined Duret's thalamic vascularization pedicles: premamillary, thalamoperforating, thalamogeniculate, choroidal and lenticulo-optic. The participation of the choroidal artery in the vascularization of the thalamus had already been recorded in a summary diagram [45] (Figure 6B).

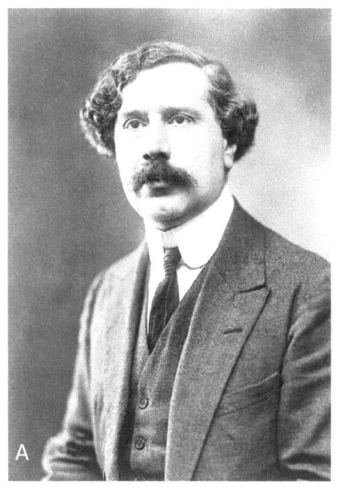 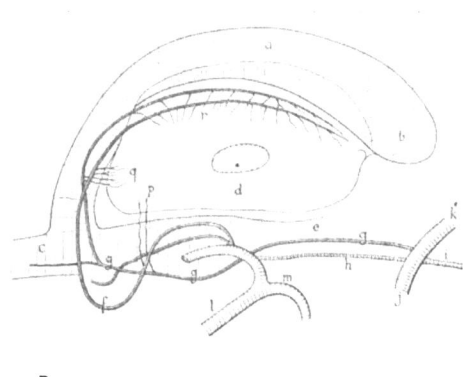

A B

Figure 6. (**A**) Charles Foix (1882–1927) (public domain). (**B**) Arterial vascularization of the human thalamus from Foix and Hillemand's work. Arterial participation of the anterior choroidal artery in the thalamus vascularization is already mentioned here (p). Reprinted from [45], used with permission.

The next stage was the study of the blood supply to the brain stem. Before this, there had been few studies addressing this question, although Duret had studied the vascularization of the medulla oblongata and its cranial nerves in 1873, and John Sebastian Bach Stopford (1888–1961) had studied the vascularization of the medulla oblongata and the pons [33,46,47].

Foix and Hillemand proposed an extraparenchymal classification of the arteries as paramedian, short circumferential, and long circumferential, which correspond to the three sections of the brain stem [48,49].

Foix also studied the anatomy of the anterior and middle cerebral arteries and their clinical syndromes [50,51]. The distribution territories of both arteries were different to those described by Duret, but he did not discuss the variability of the cortical arterial territories in detail. Neither did he comment on the notion introduced at the same time by the Australian Joseph Lexden Shellshear (1885–1958) claiming that the cerebral territories vary insignificantly according to the slight variations of the functional areas of the brain cortex [52].

Among these anatomical masterpieces, Foix developed only one inaccurate hypothesis, which led to many controversies: the existence of the "artère de la fossette latérale du bulbe", a circumferential artery originating from the basilar artery. He wrongly believed that this artery was responsible for lateral medullary syndrome. Foix refuted the view of Adolf Wallenberg (1862–1949), who believed the vascularisation of the lateral fossette of the medulla oblongata to be multi-arterial [49,53].

Foix tempered some inaccurate concepts, such as the existence of the lenticulo-optic arteries. Presumably out of respect for his predecessors, Duret and Charcot, Foix mentioned the lenticulo-optic arteries in his early work, but over time, this arterial pedicle had a decreasingly prominent role in his presentation of the vascularization of the thalamus. Foix increasingly doubted the existence of the arteries and ultimately denied their involvement in thalamic infarctions [51].

The relationship between anatomy and clinical signs was a constant source of interest for Foix for each of the arteries he studied, resulting in the first reliable descriptions of vascular syndromes. He re-examined certain syndromes that had already become well established, such as pontine crossed syndromes: "Were it not for fear of being accused of paradox, we could say that encountering a clear case of Millard-Gübler syndrome or Raymond-Cestan syndrome almost allows us to eliminate the diagnosis of softening... Indeed, softening of the pons obeys constant rules according to the vascular disposition." [54].

Although some of Charles Foix's innovative ideas have only recently been rediscovered, he remains the first true vascular neurologist, the first who truly understood the importance of arterial anatomy in understanding semiology [55,56].

6. Building on a Legacy

Before the advent of neuroimaging, injection studies were the most effective method to examine the brain's vascular organization. Paired with anatomo-clinical correlations, they refined the seminal works of Heubner, Beevor, Duret, and Foix.

Charles Foix's descriptions provided a solid basis for subsequent anatomical works that were corroborated and supplemented by anatomists and vascular neurologists. Among them, the Australian anatomist Andrew Arthur Abbie (1905–1976) was particularly interested in the anterior choroidal artery, situating his experiments in a phylogenetic framework [57,58].

The brainstem's arterial vascularisation and corresponding vascular syndromes were thoroughly studied by Lois A. Gillilan (1911-1991), Guy Lazorthes (1910–2014) and Henri Duvernoy (1931–2021) (Figure 7). They supplemented the extra-parenchymatal classification of brainstem arteries suggested by Foix and Hillemand with the definition of the intraprenchymatous arterial territories we use nowadays. They also specified the complex arterial organization of the pons for a better clinical understanding of its syndromes [59–61].

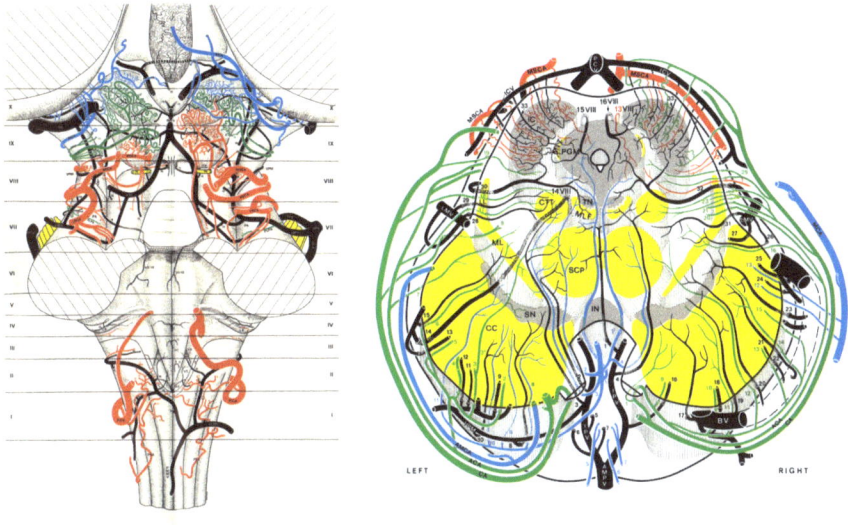

Figure 7. Diagrams of brainstem vascularization by Henri Duvernoy (1931–2021). Reprinted from [61], used with permission.

The princeps thalamus arterial supply described by Foix was also refined. Abbie formally confirmed that Duret's lenticulo-optic artery did not exist [56]. The arterial pedicles and participation of the anterior choroidal artery were confirmed by Christiaan Plets (1939–2015) [62]. The anatomical variations of the thalamic arterial pedicles were studied by Gérard Percheron (1930–2011) [63].

7. Conclusions

The question of the variability of the arterial cortical territories introduced by Beevor after the works of Heubner and Duret as well as the role of arterial anastomoses has been widely debated. The way in which anastomoses of the cortical arteries function in normal conditions compared to during a cerebral infarction was assessed by two anatomical and anatomo-pathological studies [64]. Improved techniques allowed anatomists to study microvascularization, and Duvernoy focused on the cerebral and cerebellar cortexes [65,66]. However, his magnificent studies did not completely resolve the still-debated question of the anastomoses and variability of the arterial cortical territories.

Author Contributions: Conceptualization, L.T. and J.B. Investigation L.T. and J.B. Writing—Original Draft Preparation L.T.; Writing—Review & Editing J.B.

Funding: This research received no external funding.

Acknowledgments: We would like to thank Jennifer Dobson for proofreading this manuscript.

Conflicts of Interest: The authors declare no conflict of interest.

References

1. Von Staden, H. *Herophilus: The Art of Medicine in Early Alexandria*; Cambridge University Press: Cambridge, UK, 1989.
2. Von Staden, H. The discovery of the body: Human dissection and its cultural contexts in Ancient Greece. *Yale J. Biol. Med.* **1992**, *65*, 223–241. [PubMed]
3. Nutton, V. *Ancient Medicine*; Routledge: London, UK, 2004.
4. Galen. *De usu partium*; Translation from the Greek by Margaret T. May; Cornell University Press: Ithaca, NY, USA, 1968; Volume 1, pp. 430–431.
5. Rocca, J. Galen and the Ventricular System. *J. Hist. Neurosci.* **1997**, *6*, 227–239. [CrossRef] [PubMed]
6. Olry, R. Medieval neuroanatomy: The text of Mondino dei Luzzi and the plates of Guido da Vigevano. *J. Hist. Neurosci.* **1997**, *6*, 113–123. [CrossRef] [PubMed]
7. Sudhoff, K. Ein provenzalischer anatomischer Traktat aus dem 13. Jahrhundert. In *Ein Betrag zur Geschichte der Anatomie im Mittelalter*; J.A. Barth: Leipzig, Germany, 1908.
8. Hundt, M. *Antropologium de hominis dignitate, natura, et Proprietatibus, de elementis, partibus et membris humani corporis*; Wolfgang Stöckel: Leipzig, Germany, 1501.
9. Berengarius da Carpi, J. *Commentaria cum amplissimus additionibus super anatomiam Mundini*; Hyeronimum de Benedictis: Bologne, Italy, 1521.
10. Berengarius da Carpi, J. *Isagogæ breves perlucidæ ac uberrimæ in anatomiam humani corporis*; Benedictum Hectoris: Bologne, Italy, 1523.
11. Vesalius, A. *Tabulae anatomicae Sex*; Sumptibus Ioannis Stephani Calcarensis: Venice, Italy, 1538.
12. Vesalius, A. *De humani corporis fabrica libri septem*; Ex Officina Joannis Oporini: Basle, Switzerland, 1543.
13. Lanska, D. Evolution of the myth of the human rete mirabile traced through text and illustrations in printed books: The case of Vesalius and his plagiarists. *J. Hist. Neurosci.* **2022**, *31*, 221–261. [CrossRef]
14. Willis, T. *Cerebri anatome: Cui accessit nervorum description et usus*; Tho. Roycroft: London, UK, 1664.
15. Meyer, A.; Hierrons, R. Observations on the history of the circle of Willis. *Med. Hist.* **1962**, *6*, 119–130. [CrossRef]
16. Fallopio, G. *Observationes anatomicae*; Marcum Antonium Ulmum: Venice, Italy, 1562.
17. Spigelius, A. *De humani corporis fabrica in libri decem*; Bucretius, D., Ed.; Evangelista Deuchinus: Venice, Italy, 1627.
18. Vesling, J. *Syntagma anatomicum*; Paolo Frambotto: Padua, Italy, 1647.
19. Wepfer, J.J. *Observationes anatomicae ex cadaveribus eorum, quos sustulit apoplexia cum exercitatione de ejus loco affect*; JK Suter: Schaffhausen, Switzerland, 1658.
20. Pranghoffer, S. "It could be seen more clearly in cnreasonable animals than in humans": The representation of the rete mirabile in early modern anatomy. *Med. Hist.* **2009**, *53*, 561–586. [CrossRef]
21. De Vieussens, R. *Neurographia hoc est, omnium corporis humani nervorum simul & cerebri, medullaeque spinalis descriptio anatomica*; Joannem Certier: Lyon, France, 1684.

22. Ridley, H. *The Anatomy of the Brain, Containing Its Mechanism and Physiology*; Together with Some New Discoveries and Corrections of Ancient and Modern Authors upon That Subject; Smith and Walford: London, UK, 1695.
23. Vicq d'Azyr, F. *Traité d'Anatomie et de Physiologie (Tome Premier)*; Didot: Paris, France, 1786.
24. Soemmering, S.T. *Vom Baue des menschlichen Körpers*; Barrentrapp und Werner: Frankfurt am Main, Germany, 1791–1796.
25. Rochoux, J.A. *Recherches sur l'Apoplexie*; Méquignon-Marvis: Paris, France, 1814.
26. Rostan, L. *Recherches sur le ramollissement du cerveau*; Bechet: Paris, France, 1823.
27. Lobstein, J.F. *Traité d'anatomie pathologique*; Levrault: Paris, France, 1829.
28. Virchow, R. Ueber die acute Entzündung der Arterien. *Arch. Pathol. Anat.* **1847**, *1*, 272–378. [CrossRef]
29. Heubner, O. Zur Topographie des Ernährungsgebiete der einzelnen Hirnarterien. *Cent. Die Med. Wiss.* **1872**, *52*, 817–821.
30. Walusinski, O.; Courivaud, P. Henry Duret (1849–1921): A Surgeon and Forgotten Neurologist. *Eur. Neuology* **2014**, *72*, 193–202. [CrossRef]
31. Duret, H. Recherches anatomiques sur la circulation de l'encéphale. *Arch. Physiol. Norm. Pathol.* **1874**, *6*, 60–91.
32. Duret, H. Recherches anatomiques sur la circulation de l'encéphale. III Artères corticales ou des circonvolutions cérébrales. *Arch. Physiol. Norm. Pathol.* **1874**, *6*, 316–353.
33. Duret, H. Sur la distribution des artères nourricières du bulbe rachidien. *Arch. Physiol. Norm. Pathol.* **1873**, *5*, 97–114.
34. Paciaroni, M.; Bogousslavsky, J. How did stroke become of interest to neurologists? *Neurology* **2009**, *73*, 724–728. [CrossRef] [PubMed]
35. Charcot, J.M. *Leçons sur les localisations dans les maladies du cerveau*; 5e à 8e leçons; Delahaye: Paris, France, 1876.
36. Kolisko, A. *Über die Beziehung der Arteria choroidea anterior zum hinteren Schenkel der inneren Kapsel des Gehirnes*; Alfred Hödler: Wien, Austria, 1891.
37. Ayer, J.B.; Aitken, H.F. Note on the arteries of the corpus striatum. *Boston Med. Surg. J.* **1907**, *156*, 768–771. [CrossRef]
38. Aitken, H.F. *A Report on the Circulation of the Lobar Ganglia Made to Dr. James B. Ayer*; Fort Hill Press: Harvard, MA, USA, 1909.
39. Duret, H. Revue critique de quelques recherches récentes sur la circulation cérébrale. *Encéphale* **1910**, *1*, 7–27.
40. Compston, A. From the archives. The cerebral arterial supply. By Charles E Beevor MD, FRCP. Brain 1908, 30, 403–425. *Brain* **2013**, *136*, 362–367. [CrossRef]
41. Beevor, C.E. On the Distribution of the Different Arteries Supplying the Human Brain. *Philos. Trans. R. Soc. London Ser. B* **1909**, *200*, 1–55.
42. Beevor, C.E. The cerebral arterial supply. *Brain* **1908**, *30*, 403–425. [CrossRef]
43. Hillemand, P. Charles Foix et son oeuvre 1882–1927. *Clio Med.* **1976**, *11*, 269–287.
44. Foix, C.; Masson, A. Le syndrome de l'artère cérébrale postérieure. *Presse Med.* **1923**, *31*, 361–365.
45. Foix, C.; Hillemand, P. Les syndromes de la région thalamique. *Presse Med.* **1925**, *33*, 113.

46. Stopford, J.S.B. The arteries of the pons and medulla oblongata. Part 1. *J. Anat. Physiol.* **1916**, *30*, 131–164.
47. Stopford, J.S.B. The arteries of the pons and medulla oblongata. Part 2. *J. Anat. Physiol.* **1916**, *30*, 256–280.
48. Foix, C.; Hillemand, P. Note sur la disposition générale des artères de l'axe encéphalique. *Compte-Rendus La Société Biol.* **1925**, *92*, 31–33.
49. Foix, C.; Hillemand, P. Les artères de l'axe encéphalique jusqu'au diencéphale inclusivement. *Rev. Neurol.* **1925**, *41*, 705–739.
50. Foix, C.; Hillemand, P. Les syndromes de l'artère cérébrale anterieure. *Encephale* **1925**, *20*, 209–232;
51. Foix, C.; Levy, M. Les ramollissements sylviens. *Rev. Neurol.* **1927**, *43*, 1–51.
52. Shellshear, J.L. A contribution to our knowledge of the arterial supply of the cerebral cortex in man. *Brain* **1927**, *50*, 236–253. [CrossRef]
53. Foix, C.; Hillemand, P.; Schalit, I. Sur le syndrome latéral du bulbe et l'irrigation du bulbe supérieur. *Rev. Neurol.* **1925**, *41*, 160–179.
54. Foix, C.; Hillemand, P. Contribution à l'étude des ramollissements protubérantiels. *Rev. Med.* **1926**, *43*, 287–305.
55. Caplan, L.R. Charles Foix—The first modern stroke neurologist. *Stroke* **1990**, *21*, 348–356. [CrossRef] [PubMed]
56. Tatu, L.; Moulin, T.; Monnier, G. The discovery of encephalic arteries. From Johann Jakob Wepfer to Charles Foix. *Cerebrovasc. Dis.* **2005**, *20*, 427–432. [CrossRef] [PubMed]
57. Abbie, A.A. The clinical significance of the anterior choroidal artery. *Brain* **1933**, *56*, 233–246. [CrossRef]
58. Abbie, A.A. The anatomy of capsular vascular disease. *Med. J. Aust.* **1937**, *2*, 564–568. [CrossRef]
59. Gillilan, L.A. The correlation of the blood supply to the human brain stem with clinical brain stem lesions. *J. Neuropathol. Exp. Neurol.* **1964**, *23*, 78–108. [CrossRef]
60. Lazorthes, G.; Poulhes, G.; Bastide, G.; Roulleau, J. Les territoires artériels du tronc cérébral. Recherches anatomiques et syndromes vasculaires. *Presse Méd.* **1958**, *91*, 2048–2051.
61. Duvernoy, H.M. *Human Brainstem Vessels*; Springer: Berlin, Germany, 1978.
62. Plets, C.; De Reuck, J.; Vander Eecken, H.; van der Bergh, R. The vascularization of the human thalamus. *Acta Neurol. Belg.* **1970**, *70*, 687–770.
63. Percheron, G. The anatomy of the arterial supply of the human thalamus and its use for the interpretation of the thalamic vascular pathology. *Z. Neurol.* **1973**, *205*, 1–13. [CrossRef]
64. Vander Eecken, H.M.; Adams, R.D. The anatomy and functional significance of the meningeal arterial anastomoses of the human brain. *J. Neuropathol. Exp. Neurol.* **1953**, *12*, 132–157. [CrossRef]
65. Duvernoy, H.M.; Delon, S.; Vannson, J.L. Cortical blood vessels of the human brain. *Brain Res. Bull.* **1981**, *7*, 519–579. [CrossRef]
66. Duvernoy, H.M.; Delon, S.; Vannson, J.L. The vascularization of the human cerebellar cortex. *Brain Res. Bull.* **1983**, *11*, 419–480. [CrossRef] [PubMed]

© 2023 by the authors. Licensee MDPI, Basel, Switzerland. This article is an open access article distributed under the terms and conditions of the Creative Commons Attribution (CC BY) license (http://creativecommons.org/licenses/by/4.0/).

The Evolving Concepts of Apoplexy and Brain Softening

Olivier Walusinski

Abstract: Paralysis, affecting motion or sensation, is a condition known from immemorial time. Apoplexy was the generic term used to indicate its cerebral origin until Wepfer established a correlation between apoplexy and cerebral haemorrhage in 1658. During the 17th and 18th centuries, its pathophysiology was discussed, and several hypotheses were suggested, but it was only during the 19th century that cerebral ischaemia and infarction concepts appeared and became recognised as the more prevalent form of stroke. This chapter deals with the history of the emergence and acknowledgment of cerebrovascular brain insult's physiopathology.

1. Early Concepts

Stroke has been recognised and described since ancient times, when it was included within the larger syndrome known as apoplexy. In 1721, Hélie Hélian (1658–?) gave this definition: "Apoplexy is a permanent, sudden numbing and affects organs under voluntary control, resulting in loss of feeling and movement whereas the pulse and breathing remain nearly in their natural state" [1]. The German Johann Jakob Wepfer (1650–1695) established the first correlation between apoplexy and cerebral haemorrhage in 1658, after having described the carotid siphon (Figure 1) [2]. In addition, he sketched out a pathophysiological framework by referring to arterial rupture as the cause of haemorrhage and a secondary obstruction of the "corpora fibrosa" in the wall.

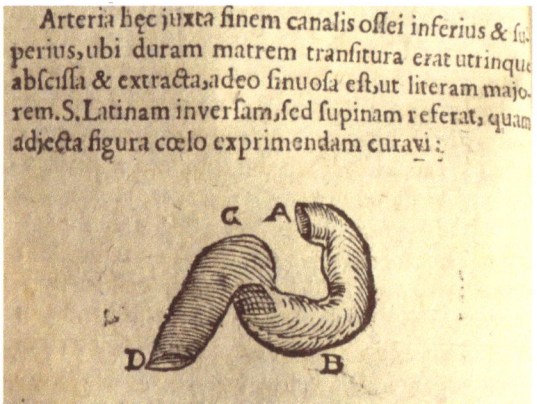

Figure 1. JJ. Wepfer described and drew the carotid siphon. Source: Photo by the author (© Photo by the author from Reference [2]; author books collection).

2. Vascular Origins Identified

In 1677, the iatromathematician François Bayle (1622–1709) in Toulouse first reviewed the various pathophysiological theories of apoplexy, such as brain compression, and then made his own proposition: Calcifications in the carotid walls explain their fragility and their propensity to break or be blocked [3]. In 1684, the English physician and anatomist Thomas Willis (1622–1675) confirmed that, with some exceptions, apoplexy was caused by an intracranial extravasation of blood. For him, the seat of apoplexy was the "callous body," by which he meant the white matter of the cerebrum [4]. He maintained that the extensive anastomoses between the large cerebral blood vessels (i.e., the circle of Willis) precluded apoplexy that was due to the obstruction of a single artery, but he did not comment on the occlusion of the smaller branches of cephalic arteries [5]. In Pisa, Domenico Mistichelli (1675–1715) demonstrated in 1709 that the side of the body contralateral to the cerebral localisation of the haemorrhage was paralysed [6].

The founding pathological anatomy work by Giovanni Battista Morgagni (1682–1771) owes much to the seventy cases of apoplexy autopsied by Théophile Bonet (1620–1689) in Geneva [7]. Bonet suggested that blood disorders ("thin" or "acid" blood) may favour the extravasation of blood from the vessels. Morgagni did not offer any new concepts, but he did suggest a classification that the Scottish William Cullen (1710–1790) took up again in 1769: sanguine, serous, traumatic, mental, atrabilious, and hydrocephalous apoplexy. The last form, described in children, brings tuberculous meningitis to mind [8]. This classification spread rapidly despite the difficulty of distinguishing between the different forms at the patient's bedside, as noted in France by Pierre Dan Delavauterie (1780–1868) in his 1807 thesis [9] and by Antoine Portal (1742–1832) in 1811 [10]. Furthermore, while the link between arterial disease and apoplexy was well established, notably by the Scottish anatomopathologist Matthew Baillie (1761–1823) [11], the origin of the serous form remained hypothetical. In 1820, John Cooke (1756–1838) considered serous apoplexy to be rare [12].

3. A Single Cause of Apoplexy, Haemorrhage

As early as 1812 in France, Jean-André Rochoux (1787–1852) [13] only recognised a single cause of apoplexy, haemorrhage, in his thesis: "It essentially consists of haemorrhage by rupture, more or less considerable, sometimes outside the brain but usually within its substance" [14].

The same year, John Cheyne (1777–1836) introduced the concept of cerebral anaemia, i.e., a reduction in cerebral flow. He did not, however, give a clear cause. In those who survived "a stroke of apoplexy," Cheyne observed a cavity filled with serous fluid in the cerebral matter after their death, indicating resorption in the blood [15]. To this inadvertent description of cerebral infarct, he added the observation of a breathing pattern characterised by alternating periods of apnoea and hyperpnoea, leading to the eponym "Cheyne–Stokes respiration" [16].

4. Cerebral Softening is More Prevalent Than Haemorrhage

In two successive works, in 1820 [17] and then in 1823, Léon Rostan (1790–1866) was the first to attempt to distinguish what he called the cerebral softening of apoplexy, that is, haemorrhagic infarct. According to Rostan, softening was the most frequent cause of hemiplegia, whereas haemorrhage was rare, but he did not fail to mention that haemorrhage may follow softening. He established this new paradigm by comparing it to gangrene in the limbs of the elderly: "The arteries of the brain are usually ossified when this organ is softened". Softening was thus a well-defined anatomopathological entity that became a disease of the vessels [18]: "The vessels that bring blood and life to the affected organ are ossified not following inflammation but by the ageing process".

5. Arterial Obstruction as the Pathogenesis

In 1824, François-Claude Lallemand (1790–1853) only saw softening "as partial inflammation of the brain" [19], which Gabriel Andral (1797–1876) was quick to contradict in 1829 [20]. Andral was of Rostan's opinion that there was a similarity with gangrene in the limbs secondary to "suspension of the circulation by arterial disease". Baillie, in the last edition of his pathological anatomy treatise in 1818 [21], had already referred to this pathophysiology.

In 1828, John Abercrombie (1780–1844) classified apoplexy into three types depending on the sudden or progressive onset, with or without coma, and with or without functional recovery. He discussed aetiologies involving either arterial spasm blocking circulation or rupture of the arterial wall. He also noted frequent calcifications in the elderly [22]. After being a proponent of the inflammatory theory developed by Lallemand, he became a proponent of Rostan after reading his book. Arterial obstruction as the pathogenesis of softening was controversial for another quarter of a century. For example, the Scottish pathologist Robert Carswell (1793–1857) subscribed to it in 1833 [23], whereas in 1843 [24], the French Maxime Durand-Fardel (1815–1899), following in the footsteps of Jean-Baptiste Bouillaud (1796–1881), maintained that inflammation played a preponderant role [25]. At the same time, Carl Rokitansky (1804–1878) in Vienna drew attention to the frequent association between hypertrophy of the left heart ventricle and apoplexy, indirectly linking arterial hypertension and cerebral haemorrhage [26].

6. Thrombosis and Embolism

In 1847, Rudolf Virchow (1821–1902) made decisive arguments confirming the vascular theory of softening by introducing the concepts of thrombosis and embolism: "These clots never originate in the local circulation but are torn off at a distance and carried along in the blood stream as far as they can go" [27]. In fact, Virchow brought back the notions of clots and arteriosclerosis already proposed (but without garnering much attention) by Jean-Frédéric Lobstein (1777–1835) in Strasbourg in 1829 [28]. In 1852, William Senhouse Kirkes (1822–1864) was the first to describe three cases of cerebral embolism after finding either clots in the right atrium or valve vegetations [29]. In his thesis defended on 07 March 1862 [30], Étienne Lancereaux (1829–1910) provided a lengthy bibliography of European authors confirming the thromboembolic theory of brain softening.

In 1866, Jean-Baptiste-Vincent Laborde (1830–1903), a student of Rostan, used a microscope to show that softening is a non-inflammatory, organic phenomenon, secondary to damage of the capillary walls in brain tissue and calcareous incrustations. In another attempt in 1866, Adrien Proust (1834–1903) suggested that softening indicated a functional defect of the circle of Willis by the obstruction of backup circulatory routes [31].

7. Experimental Demonstration

Ferdinand Cohn (1828–1898), who became a pioneer in bacteriology, reported numerous experiments in the treatise of von Rokitansky that were conducted in animals involving ligation or injection of inert bodies to block arteries and observe the cerebral lesions downstream [32]. In 1866, Jules Cotard (1840–1889), a student of Jean-Martin Charcot (1825–1893), and Jean-Louis Prévost (1838–1927), a student of Alfred Vulpian (1826–1887), repeated these experiments on rabbits and confirmed that the injection of fine powder (lycopodium spores) or coarser substances (tobacco seeds) triggered different forms of paralysis that varied according to the size of the occlusion and depending on whether it was proximal or peripheral. Tobacco seeds blocked the middle cerebral artery and caused a non-haemorrhagic pinkish softening, comparable to the softening found during the autopsies of their patients. They described the changes over time in the lesions, first involving "anaemic" signs and later infiltrations of blood (hyperaemia) [33].

8. Charcot, Duret, and Foix Lay the Foundations of Current Vascular Neurology

The same year, Charcot recorded the observation of a hemiplegic patient. He proposed a complete explanation of the pathophysiology of cerebral infarction and described the ulceration of an atheromatous plaque at the intima of an artery, on which a clot aggregates, blocks the vessel, or flows downstream as an embolus, causing cerebral ischaemia and parenchymal lesions (Figure 2). Using the term "cholestérine" (cholesterin), the name of cholesterol at the time, he identified the biological nature of atheromatous plaques and made detailed drawings [34].

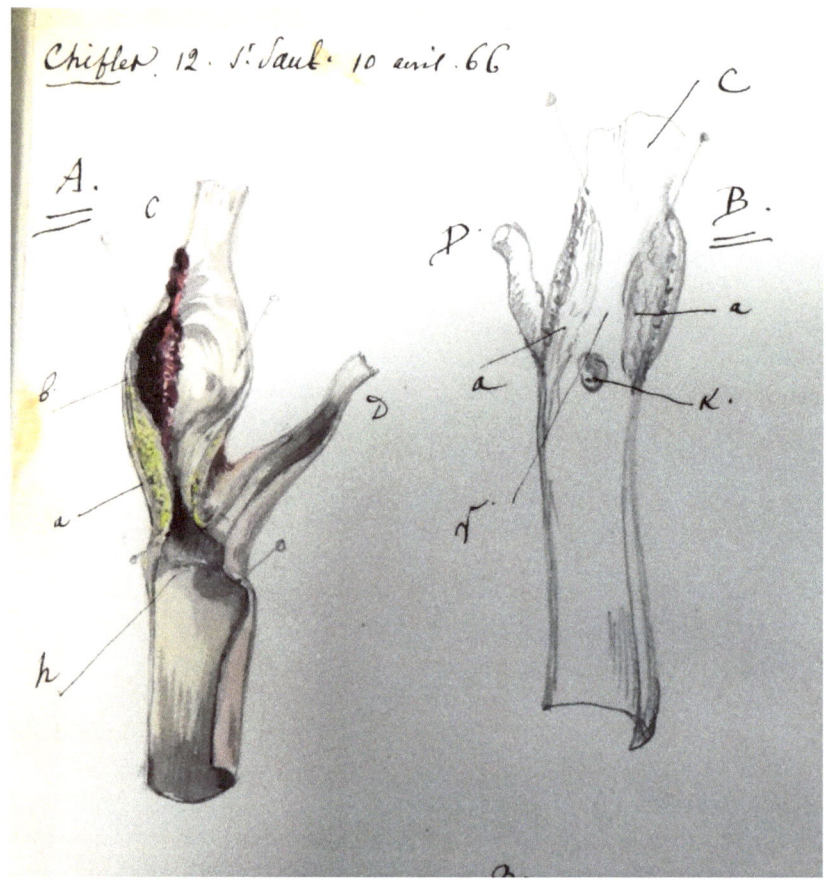

Figure 2. Drawing by Charcot of the ulceration of an atheromatous plaque of the carotide. Bibliothèque Charcot (Source: © Photo by the author; Charcot Library, Sorbonne Université, used with permission).

The decisive step occurred in Charcot's laboratory in 1874. Henri Duret (1849–1921), using injections of coloured gelatine, described the distribution of "supply arteries" of the brainstem, then the cortex, correlating the irrigated territories, infarcted areas, and secondary neurological deficits (Figure 3) [35,36]. Julius Cohnheim (1839–1884) had already proposed this pathophysiology in humans in 1872, more theoretically, and introduced the concept of ischaemic necrosis which he distinguished from haemorrhagic infarct [37].

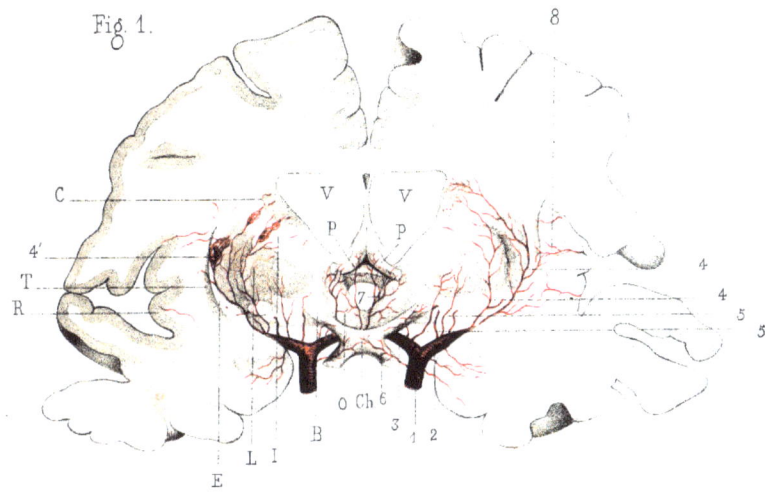
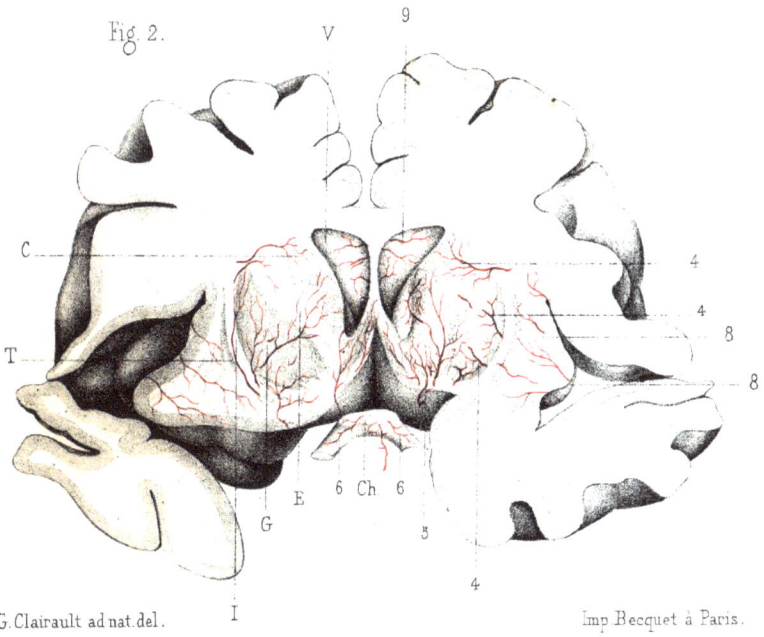

Figure 3. Drawing by Duret the distribution of the basal ganglia's arteries. (Source: Photo by the author from Ref [35]; Author books collection).

Finally, Charles Foix (1882–1927) [38], the first real vascular neurologist, described the clinical syndromes involving each sylvian [39] and basilar [40] arterial territory between 1923 and his death in 1927, ushering in the contemporary era of vascular pathology.

Funding: This research received no external funding.

Acknowledgments: Many thanks to Julien Bogousslavsky, Jacques Poirier and Hubert Déchy for their proofreading and to Anna Fitzgerald for her translation.

Conflicts of Interest: The author has no conflicts of interest to declare.

References

1. Helian, H. *Dictionnaire du Diagnostic ou l'art de Connoître les Maladies et les Distinguer Exactement les unes des Autres*; Chez Vincent: Paris, France, 1721.
2. Wepfer, J.J. *Observationes Anatomicae, ex Cadaveribus Eorum, quos Sustulit Apoplexia, cum Exercitatione de eius Loco Affecto*; Joh Caspari Suteri: Schaffhausen, Switzerland, 1658.
3. Bayle, F. *Tractatus de Apoplexia: In Quo Hujus Affectionis Causa Penitius Inquiritur & Curatio Exponitur Ex Doctrina Hippocratis*; Guillemette, B.: Tolosæ, France, 1677.
4. Willis, T. *Dr Willis's Practice of Physick, Being the Whole Works of That Renowned and Famous Physician: Containing These Eleven Several Treatises. Two Discourses Concerning the Soul of Brutes. Wherein Most of the Diseases Belonging to the Body of Man Are Treated of, with Excellent Methods and Receipts for the Cure of the Same*; Dring, T.; Harper, C.; Leigh, J.: London, UK, 1684.
5. Tatu, L.; Moulin, T.; Monnier, G. The discovery of encephalic arteries. From Johann Jacob Wepfer to Charles Foix. *Cerebrovasc. Dis.* **2005**, *20*, 427–432. [CrossRef] [PubMed]
6. Finger, S. *Origins of Neuroscience: A History of Explorations into Brain Function*. Oxford University Press: New York, USA, 1994.
7. Schutta, H.S.; Howe, H.M. Seventeenth century concepts of "apoplexy" as reflected in Bonet's "Sepulchretum". *J. Hist. Neurosci.* **2006**, *15*, 250–268. [CrossRef]
8. Cullen, W. *Synopsis nosologiae methodicae in usum studiosorum. Editio altera. In Quarta Parte Emendata et Adjectis Morborum Specierus Aucta*; Kincaid A., Creech, W.; Johnston, W.; Cadell, T.; Murray, J.; Dilly, E.: Edinburgi, UK, 1772.
9. Dan Delavauterie, P. *Dissertation sur L'apoplexie Considérée Spécialement Comme l'effet d'une Phlegmasie de la Substance Cérébrale*; Thèse n°68, impr.; Didot Jeune: Paris, France, 1807.
10. Portal, A. *Observations sur la nature et le Traitement de L'apoplexie et sur les Moyens de la Prévenir*; Chez Crochard: Paris, France, 1811.
11. Baillie, M. *The Morbid Anatomy of Some of the Most Important Parts of the Human Body*; Johnson J.: London, UK, 1793.
12. Cooke, J. On Apoplexy including Apoplexia hydrocephalica. In *Treatise on Nervous Diseases*; Cooke, J., Ed.; Longman, Hurst, Rees, Orme, Brown: London, UK, 1820.
13. Walusinski, O. Jean-André Rochoux (1787–1852), a physician philosopher at the dawn of vascular neurology. *Rev. Neurol (Paris).* **2017**, *173*, 532–541. [CrossRef] [PubMed]
14. Rochoux, J.A. *Propositions sur L'apoplexie*; Thèse n°73, impr.; Didot Jeune: Paris, France, 1812.

15. Cheyne, J. *Cases of Apoplexy and Lethargy with Observations Upon the Comatose Diseases*; Thomas Underwood: London, UK; Adam Black: Edinburgh, UK; Walter Duncan: Glasgow, UK; Gilbert & Hodges: Dublin, Ireland, 1812.
16. Cheyne, J. A case of apoplexy in which the fleshy part of the heart was converted into fat. *Dublin Hosp. Rep.* **1818**, *2*, 216–223.
17. Rostan, L. *Recherches sur une Maladie encore peu Connue qui a reçu le nom de Ramollissement du Cerveau*; Béchet et Crevot: Paris, France, 1820.
18. Poirier, J.; Desrouesné, C. La neurologie à l'assistance publique et en particulier à La Salpêtrière avant Charcot, l'exemple de Rostan et du ramollissement cérébral. *Rev. Neurol (Paris)* **2000**, *156*, 607–615. [PubMed]
19. Lallemand, F.C. *Recherches Anatomo-Pathologiques sur L'encéphale et ses Dépendances*; Béchet Jeune: Paris, France, 1824–1830.
20. Andral, G. *Précis D'anatomie-Pathologique*; Gabon: Paris, France, 1829.
21. Baillie, M. *The Morbid Anatomy of Some the Most Important Parts of the Human Body*; Nicol, J, &W.: London, UK, 1818.
22. Abercrombie, J. *Pathological and Practical Researches on Diseases of the Brain and the Spinal Cord*; Waugh and Innes: Edinburgh, UK, 1828.
23. Carswell, R. Softening. In *The Cyclopædia of Practical Medicine: Comprising Treatises on the Nature and Treatment of Diseases, Materia Medica and Therapeutics, Medical Jurisprudence, etc.*; Forbes, J., Ed.; Lea & Blanchard: Philadelphia, PA, USA, 1833–1835.
24. Durand-Fardel, M. *Traité du Ramollissement du Cerveau*; Baillière, J.-B.: Paris, France, 1843.
25. Bouillaud, J.B. *Traité Clinique et Physiologique de L'encéphalite ou Inflammation du Cerveau et de Ses Suites: Telles que le Ramollissement, la Suppuration, les Abcès, les Tubercules, le Squirrhe, le Cancer, etc.*; Baillière, J.-B.: Paris, France, 1825.
26. Rokitansky von, K. *Handbuch der Speciellen Pathologischen Anatomie*; Braumüller & Seidel: Wien, Austria, 1842.
27. Virchow, R. Über die akute Entzündung der Artérien. *Arch. Für Pathol. Anat. Und Physiol. Und Für Klin. Med. (Virchow Arch.)* **1847**, *1*, 272–378. [CrossRef]
28. Lobstein, J.F. *Traité D'anatomie Pathologique*; Chez Levrault F.G.: Paris et Strasbourg, France, 1829.
29. Kirkes, W.S. Detachment of fibrinous deposits from the interior of the heart, and their mixture with the circulating blood. *Med.-Chir. Trans. Lond.* **1852**, *35*, 281–324. [CrossRef] [PubMed]
30. Lancereaux, E. *De la Thrombose et de L'embolie Cérébrales Considérées Principalement Dans Leurs Rapports avec le Ramollissement du Cerveau*; Thèse n°39, impr.; Rignoux: Paris, France, 1862.
31. Proust, A. *Des Différentes formes de Ramollissement du Cerveau*; Asselin: Paris, France, 1866.
32. Rokitansky von, K. *Handbuch der Pathologischen Anatomie*; Braumüller & Seidel: Wien, Austria, 1855–1861.
33. Prévost, J.L.; Cotard, J. Études physiologiques et pathologiques sur le ramollissement cérébral. *Comptes Rendus Des Séances Et Mémoires De La Société De Biol.* **1866**, *2*, 49–53.
34. Walusinski, O. Charcot and Cholesterin. *Eur. Neurol* **2019**, *81*, 309–318. [CrossRef] [PubMed]

35. Duret, H. Recherches anatomiques sur la circulation de l'encéphale. *Arch. De Physiol. Norm. Et Pathol.* **1874**, *6*, 60–91.
36. Walusinski, O.; Courrivaud, P. Henry Duret (1849–1921): A surgeon and forgotten neurologist. *Eur. Neurol* **2014**, *72*, 193–202. [CrossRef] [PubMed]
37. Cohnheim, J. *Untersuchungen Über die Embolischen Processe*; Hirschwald: Berlin, Germany, 1872.
38. Caplan, L.R. Charles Foix, the first modern stroke neurologist. *Stroke* **1990**, *21*, 348–356. [CrossRef] [PubMed]
39. Foix, C.; Levy, M. Les ramollissements sylviens. *Rev. Neurol (Paris)* **1927**, *43*, 1–51.
40. Foix, C.; Masson, A. Le syndrome de l'artère cérébrale postérieure. *La Presse Médicale* **1923**, *32*, 361–365.

© 2023 by the author. Licensee MDPI, Basel, Switzerland. This article is an open access article distributed under the terms and conditions of the Creative Commons Attribution (CC BY) license (http://creativecommons.org/licenses/by/4.0/).

Introduction to the Terms Arteriosclerosis, Thrombosis and Embolism

Jukka Putaala

Abstract: Arteriosclerosis as a medical term has its origins in the 18th century and refers to "hardening of the arteries" and is composed of two words, arterio and sclerosis. Arterio is derived from the Latinized form of the Greek word arteria, which originally meant "windpipe" or "an artery". Sclerosis refers to "morbid hardening of the tissues" and -osis is a Greek suffix meaning "a state of disease". The term thrombosis has its origins in the Greek word thrombos, meaning "lump, piece, clot of blood, curd of milk". The term was first used to describe venous thrombosis. The first well-documented case of deep venous thrombosis appeared during the Middle Ages, and the major pathologic mechanisms of the disease were discovered by the middle of the 19th century, recapitulated by the German physician and pathologist Virchow. He realized that a venous thrombus can dislodge from its origins and travel through the blood stream and cause the blockade of vessels of other organs, hence also the term embolism.

1. Arteriosclerosis, Arteriolosclerosis, and Atherosclerosis

Arteriosclerosis as a medical term refers to "hardening of the arteries" and is composed of two words, arterio and sclerosis. Arterio is derived from the Latinized form of the Greek word arteria, which originally meant "windpipe" or "an artery". Sclerosis refers to "morbid hardening of the tissues" and -osis is a Greek suffix meaning "a state of disease". In current textbook classifications, arteriosclerosis refers to an overarching generic term with hardening and thickening of the arterial wall and loss of elasticity as the main underlying pathologic processes. The three distinct types of arteriosclerotic pathology include atherosclerosis, arteriolosclerosis, and Mönckeberg's medial calcific sclerosis [1].

The terminology used to describe lesions related to arteriosclerosis has its origins in the 18th century. The Greek term atheroma was first used in 1755 by Swiss anatomist Albrecht van Haller (1708–1777) to describe a space filled with gruel-like material [2]. The German-born French pathologist and surgeon Jean Frédéric Martin Lobstein (1777–1835) first used the term arteriosclerosis in 1833 to depict calcified arterial lesions [3]. For the term arteriolosclerosis, credit is given to English physician George Johnson (1818–1896), who described thickening of arterioles of the kidney in 1852 [4]. Mönckeberg's medical calcific sclerosis was named after German pathologist Johann Georg Mönckeberg (1877–1925) in 1903 [5]. Finally, the term atherosclerosis was first mentioned in the literature apparently by another German pathologist, Felix Marchand (1846–1928), in 1904 [6]. It should be noted that although the terminology describing arteriosclerosis is relatively young, the first described lesions of arteriosclerosis are in fact thousands of years old, as depicted by the Swiss-born British experimental pathologist and bacteriologist, Sir Marc Armand Ruffer (1859–1917), in his examinations on the histology of Egyptian mummies [7].

2. Thrombosis

The term thrombosis has its origins in the Greek word thrombos, meaning "lump, piece, clot of blood, curd of milk". The term was first used to describe venous thrombosis. The first well-documented case of deep venous thrombosis appeared during the Middle Ages, and the major pathologic mechanisms of the disease were discovered by the middle of the 19th century. The German physician and pathologist, Rudolph Ludwig Carl Virchow (1821–1902), also known as the "the father of modern pathology" first recapitulated the pathophysiology of thrombosis in 1858 describing the three common predisposing factors for the condition (the Virchow's triad): (1) damage to the endothelial lining of the vessel wall; (2) a hypercoagulable state, and (3) arterial or venous blood stasis [8].

3. Embolism

Virchow realized that a venous thrombus can dislodge from its origins and travel through the blood stream and cause the blockade of vessels of other organs. He stated that "The detachment of larger or smaller fragments from the end of the softening thrombus which are carried along by the current of blood and driven into remote vessels. This gives rise to the very frequent process on which I have bestowed the name of Embolia" [9]. Hence, the term embolism is also credited to Virchow, pointing to sudden obstruction of a blood vessel by an embolus. Virchow depicted two types of thrombi associated with pulmonary embolism, one that has origins in a systemic vein and embolizes to the lung and another, that arises in the pulmonary artery distal to the embolus due to blood flow stagnation. The etymological origins of these terms arise from the Greek term embolus, denoting "peg, stopper; anything pointed so as to be easily thrust in" or also "a tongue (of land), beak (of a ship)". Furthermore, another Greek word, emballein, meant "to insert, throw in, invade".

Interestingly, the first description of cardiac embolism was by a neurologist, the British Sir William Gowers (1945–1915). He described simultaneous emboli in the brain and retina, spleen and kidneys, and concluded that the emboli had originated from the left atrial appendage, which contained blood clots [10].

Funding: This research received no external funding.

Conflicts of Interest: The author declares no conflict of interest.

References

1. Kumar, V.; Abbas, A.K.; Aster, J.C. *Robbins Basic Pathology*, 10th ed.; Elsevier: Amsterdam, The Netherlands, 2017.
2. Schwartz, C.J.; Mitchell, J.R. The morphology, terminology and pathogenesis of arterial plaques. *Postgrad. Med. J.* **1962**, *38*, 25–34. [CrossRef] [PubMed]

3. Lobstein, J.F. *Traité d'anatomie pathologique*; Levrault: Paris, France, 1833.
4. Johnson, G. 1. On certain points in the Anatomy and Pathology of Bright's Disease of the Kidney. 2. On the Influence of the Minute Blood-vessels upon the Circulation. *Med. Chir. Trans.* **1868**, *51*, 57–78.3. [CrossRef] [PubMed]
5. Mönckeberg, J.G. Über die reine Mediaverkalkung der Extremitätenarterien und ihr Verhalten zur Arteriosklerose. *Virchows Arch.* **1903**, *171*, 141–167. [CrossRef]
6. Marchand, F. Über arteriosklerose (athero-sklerose). *Verhandl. D Kongr. F Inn. Med.* **1904**, *21*, 23–59.
7. Ruffer, M.A. On arterial lesions found in Egyptian mummies (1580 BC–525 AD). *J. Pathol. Bacteriol.* **1911**, *15*, 453–462. [CrossRef]
8. Virchow, R. *Die Cellularpathologie in ihrer Begründung auf physiologische und pathologische Gewebelehre*; August Hirschwald: Berlin, Germany, 1858.
9. Murray, T.J.; Huth, E.J. (Eds.) *Medicine in Quotations: Views of Health and Disease Through the Ages*, 2nd ed.; American College of Physicians: Philadelphia, PA, USA, 2006; p. 115.
10. Gowers, W.R. On a case of simultaneous embolism of centrai retinal and middle cerebral arteries. *Lancet* **1875**, *106*, 794–796. [CrossRef]

© 2023 by the author. Licensee MDPI, Basel, Switzerland. This article is an open access article distributed under the terms and conditions of the Creative Commons Attribution (CC BY) license (http://creativecommons.org/licenses/by/4.0/).

The Turning Point in Stroke Investigation for Neurologists

Maurizio Paciaroni and Julien Bogousslavsky

Abstract: Investigation into stroke was not at all expedient; in fact, stroke was never a field of critical interest for either the Salptrière or Pitìe Schools, which were attended by Vulpian and Charcot. The results from the few studies on the subject were carried out by sole researchers, including Rostan, Rochoux, Dechambre and Durand-Fardel. Subsequently, interest was first expressed by the leading pathologists, including Rokitansky and Virchow. This came upon the heels of the development of clinical–topographic correlation studies carried out by Déjerine, Marie and Foix, the latter of whom was the father of modern clinical stroke research.

1. The History of Brain Softening and Apoplexia

By comparing clinical features with autopsy, Giovanni Battista Morgagni [1] (1682–1771) laid the foundations of clinical anatomic studies in stroke, utilizing the classification of "sanguineous" (hemorrhagic) vs. "serous" (non-hemorrhagic) apoplexy. He assigned to the latter category cases that probably corresponded to infarction or edema. Subsequently, in 1814, Jean André Rochoux [2] (1787–1852) claimed that apoplexy was always the result of bleeding. Apoplexy described either the lesion (hemorrhage) or the symptoms (loss of movement and sensation). In his monograph, Rochoux also introduced the term "ramollissement" (softening) into the field of stroke care. Later, Léon Rostan (1790–1866) (Figure 1) introduced "spontaneous cerebral softening" as a body separate from encephalitis and apoplexy. However, Rostan did not adopt this. Instead, he regarded it as being similar to hemorrhagic stroke in pathological terms. Specifically, Rostan reported that pathologic and clinical features of brain softening differed from apoplexy in that the former was fatal. The definition of brain softening was harshly contested by Francois Broussais, Lallemand and Calmeil, who claimed that it was due to an "inflammation" and thus should be called encephalitis. Conversely, the ideas of Rostan were embraced by Carswell in England (1835), Abercrombie in Scotland (1836) and Andral in France (1827, 1840). While Rostan had suggested a link between a condition of the arteries (ossification) and parenchymatous lesions in his 1823 "Recherches sur les ramollissements du cerveau", these lesions were not correlated with vessel stenosis. It was in 1856 when Virchow revisited this hypothesis, [3] and the studies of Adrien Proust (1862), Vincent Laborde (1866) and Jean Louis Prévost and Jules Cotard in France (1865). These observations suggested that arterial occlusions and diminished blood flow to brain regions were the cause of softening, and these lesions were infarctions following Cohnheim's [4] hypothesis.

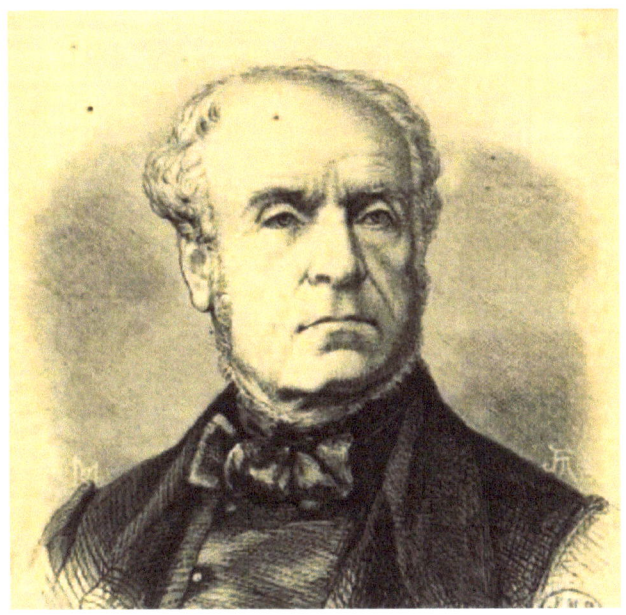

Figure 1. Léon Rostan (1790–1866). Source: Reprinted and used with permission from Olivier Walusinski (courtesy).

2. The Coining of Arteriosclerosis, Thrombosis, and Embolism

Rudolf Virchow [3] (1821–1902) was the pioneer in that he was the first to describe arterial thrombosis and embolism. This resulted from an observation he made of the interaction between blood flow and arterial walls. Specifically, he hypothesized that blocking blood flow to any major organ would result in something he later named "ischemia". At the age of 27, he was able to prove that masses in vessels would provoke something he called a "thrombosis". To better explain the underling process leading to a thrombosis, he borrowed the term "arteriosclerosis", from Lobstein, who coined it in 1829 [5]. Additionally, he is known for the fact that he was able to demonstrate that sections of a thrombosis would often flake off arterial walls and travel throughout the circulation. We know this as an embolism. Furthermore, Virchow [6] was the first to report that a local embolism can be caused by clots of heart origin in patients who had had lower limbs gangrene. He wrote that similar events in the brain may lead to cerebral softening.

Virchow was the mentor of Julius Cohnheim (1839–1884) who was the author of the term "cerebral infarct", a synonym for stroke. Cohnheim carried out experiments on arterial injection of wax globules, in which he embolized a frog's tongue. These types of embolization can lead to either no injury, or two kinds of lesions, which for over a century have been defined as "ischemic necrosis" and "hemorrhagic infarct" [4].

Karl von Rokitansky [7] (1804–1878) was responsible for a great scientific feat in the 1840s. He described that some "apoplexies" were primarily due to an enlargement of the right ventricle, whereas according to Rokitansky, hemorrhage may have been associated with hypertrophy of the left ventricle and, therein, an "impulse"; in that era, the effects of high blood pressure were not fully understood.

3. Atherosclerotic Carotid Disease: Its Evolution

After Virchow, the term carotid disease would be used to describe patients with certain combinations of eyesight loss and focal paralysis. In this regard, in 1872, Adolf Kussmaul [8] (1822–1902) and, in 1881, Franz Penzoldt [9] (1849–1927) both reported on carotid artery thrombosis in the neck region of patients afflicted with ipsilateral eye blindness [8] and contralateral hemiplegia [9].

Up until this period, the term cerebral embolism was considered to be a synonym of an embolism originating from the heart. An extracranial artery source was rarely considered up until the early 1960s. In fact, it had been assumed that arterial disease interested intracranial vessels, although Hans Chiari [10] (1851–1916) in 1905 had suggested there might be a link between extracranial carotid disease and stroke. Indeed, he observed a thrombus superimposed on ulcerated carotid plaques in 7 out of 400 autopsies. Four of these seven cases had had cerebral embolisms. This led him to suggest that thrombotic material had broken away from the observed carotid plaques and had traveled to the brain.

In 1914, James Ramsay Hunt [11] (1874–1937) suggested that an obstruction of carotid arteries could determine a "cerebral intermittent claudication". Moreover, he emphasized "the occurrence of unilateral vascular changes, pallor or atrophy of the optic disk with contralateral hemiplegia ('optico-cerebral syndrome') with carotid occlusion".

4. The Introduction of Lacunar Infarction

Used for the first time in 1838 by Amédé Dechambre [12] (1812–1886), the term lacune described a small cavity that remained after a small stroke. Subsequently, in 1843, Charles Louis Maxime Durand-Fardel [13] (1815–1899) (Figure 2) provided a more detailed explanation by defining a lacune as a small cavity in the brain "without any change in consistency or color from which it was possible to remove a little cellular tissue containing very small vessels with a thin forcep". For the next five decades, no advances were made in this field. Then, Pierre Marie (1853–1940), a pupil of Charcot, published a paper entitled "Des foyer lacunaires de désintégration et les différents autres états cavitaires du cerveau" in 1901. In this paper, he concluded that lacunes were small softenings caused by atherosclerosis. Marie also observed that lacunes tended to be asymptomatic, but "that hemiplegia in old people was more often due to cerebral lacunes than to hemorrhage or softening". During the early 20th century, all published articles on cerebral lacunes were in agreement with Marie's definition.

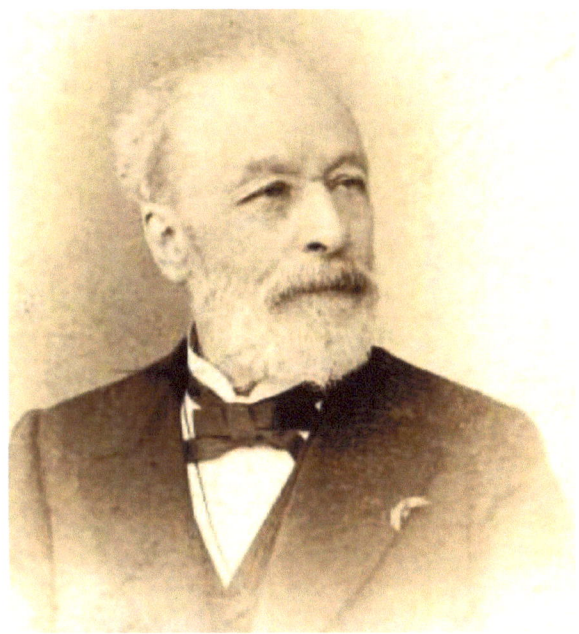

Figure 2. Charles Louis Maxime Durand-Fardel (1815–1899). Source: Reprinted and used with permission from Olivier Walusinski (courtesy).

In the 1960s, Charles Miller Fisher [14] described what he thought to be a more specific pathology of the penetrating arteries, lipohyalinosis or microatheroma, both of which lead to a characteristic of end-artery pattern vascular supply. Additionally, he suggested returning to Durand-Fardel's original definition of the term lacune, a "small, deep cerebral infarct".

5. 19th Century Clinical–Anatomic Model

By the mid-19th century, neurology had already been recognized as a medical field. However, Joseph Babinski (1857–1932), one of the most famous neurologists of this period, wrote 288 papers, with only 4 dealing in some way with stroke. Other pathologies interested researchers more. From the 19th century, clinical–anatomic methods had been disseminated throughout Europe, but it was only a bit later that clinicians began investigating an association between arterial vascularization, brain lesions and corresponding clinical features. It was, in fact, Jean-Martin Charcot (1825–1893) who taught anatomic pathology prior to having been appointed to the first chair of neurology in the world. The work of Charcot is widely recognized for its impact on neurology and psychology, but his contribution to vascular neurology remained small.

It was the description of specific brainstem syndromes, including reports by August Millard and Adolph Gubler (1856) [15,16], Achille Foville (1858) [17], Hermann David Weber (1863) [18], Moritz Benedikt (1889) [19], Adolf Wallenberg

(1901) [20], Joseph Babinski and Jean Nageotte (1902) [21] and Henri Claude (1912) [22], that lead to a great awakening. Likewise, Joseph Jules Déjerine [23] (1849–1917) (Figure 3) reported on clinical findings in stroke patients when he described, for the first time, the thalamic syndrome with Gustave Roussy.

The end of the 19th century marked the advent of the first generation of "vascular neurologists". Among these were Charles Foix [24–27] (1882–1927), a pupil of Marie, who exhibited a particular interest in cerebrovascular events. Foix is considered to be the first vascular neurologist due to his work on the patterns of brain infarction in the middle, anterior and posterior cerebral arteries and the anterior choroidal arteries [24–27]. Foix concentrated on clinical–anatomic studies, with the aim of discovering correlations between any lesion topography and clinical dysfunction. Therein, the interest in stroke gradually—though slowly—increased throughout the 20th century, especially in the 1940s and the 1950s, when the first diagnostic and therapeutic approaches of stroke were introduced. In the 1960s, Fisher described that a thromboembolic mechanism underlies most ischemic strokes and that the source of thrombus might be the heart or a proximal arterial lesion. However, it was only in the 1970s that stroke became a major research field of neurology, and this was due to results from clinical trials on anticoagulant use after ischemic stroke [28] and the first clinical trial on carotid endarterectomy [29,30].

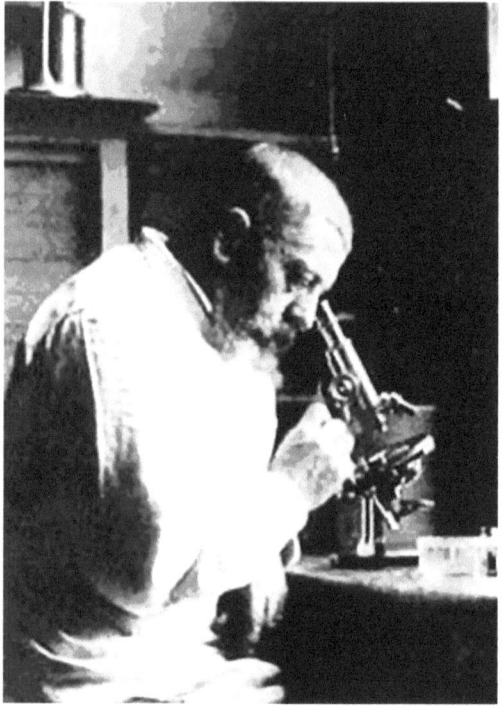

Figure 3. Joseph Jules Déjerine (1849–1917) by E. Gauckler (Masson et Cle, 1922). Source: Reprinted and used with permission from Olivier Walusinski (courtesy).

In conclusion, without the development of clinical–anatomic correlation studies at the turn of the 19th century, stroke would not have become known as a brain condition worthy of specific research. The priceless accumulation of knowledge over centuries on cerebrovascular events was the result of painstaking and courageous work on the part of single pioneers.

Author Contributions: Both Authors have drafted the work or substantively revised it and have approved the submitted version. All authors have read and agreed to the published version of the manuscript.

Funding: This review received no external funding.

Conflicts of Interest: The authors declare no conflict of interest.

References

1. Morgagni, G.B. *De Sedibus et Causis Morborum per Anatomen Indigatis Libri Quinque*; Typographica Remondiana: Venice, Italy, 1761.
2. Rochoux, J.A. *Recherches sur l'Apoplexie*; Forgotten Books: Paris, France, 1814.
3. Virchow, R.L.K. *Gesammelte Abhandlungen zur wissenschaftlichen Medizin*; Meidinger Sohn & Co.: Frankfurt, Germany, 1856; pp. 219–732.
4. Cohnheim, J. *Untersuchungen Ueber die Embolischen Prozesse*; Hirschwald: Berlin, Germany, 1872.
5. Lobstein, J.F.M. *Traité d'Anatomie Pathologique*; Levrault: Paris, France, 1829.
6. Virchow, R.L.K. Ueber die acute Entzündung der Arterien. *Arch. Pathol. Anat.* **1847**, *1*, 272–378. [CrossRef]
7. von Rokitansky, C. *A Manual of Pathological Anatomy (1824–1844)*; Sydenham Society: London, UK, 1856; Volume III, pp. 399–419.
8. Kussmau, L.A. Zwei Falle von spontaner, allmaliger Verschliessung grosser Halsarterienstamme. *Dtsch Klein* **1872**, *24*, 461–465, 473–474.
9. Penzoldt, F. Ueber Thrombose (autochtone oder embolische) der Carotis. *Dtsch. Arch. Klein. Med.* **1881**, *28*, 80–93.
10. Chiari, H. Ueber Verhalten des Teilung-swinkels der Carotis communis bei der Endarteritis chronica deformans. *Verh. Dtsch. Ges. Pathol.* **1905**, *9*, 326.
11. Hunt, J.R. The role of the carotid arteries in the causation of vascular lesions of the brain, with remarks on certain special features of the symptomatology. *Am. J. Med. Sci.* **1914**, *147*, 704–713. [CrossRef]
12. Dechambre, A. Memoire sur lacurabilitéduramollissement cerebral. *Gazette Medicale de Paris* **1938**, *6*, 305–314.
13. Durand-Fardel, C.L.M. *Traité du ramollissement du cerveau*; J.B. Bailliere: Paris, France, 1843.
14. Fisher, C.M. Lacunes: Small, deep cerebral infarcts. *Neurology* **1965**, *15*, 774–784. [CrossRef]
15. Gubler, A. Alternating hemiplegia, a sign of pontine lesion, and documentation of the proof of the facial decussation. *Gaz. Hebd. Med. Chir.* 1856, *3*, 749–754, 789–792, 811–816. In *The Classical Brainstem Syndromes*; Wolf, J.K., Translator; Charles C Thomas Publishing: Springfield, IL, USA, 1971; pp. 9–24.
16. Millard, A. Correspondence. *Gaz. Hebd. Med Chir.* **1856**, *3*, 86–818. [CrossRef]

17. Foville, A. Note sur une paralysie peu connue de certains muscles de l'oeil. *Bull. Soc. Anat. Paris* **1858**, *3*, 393–405.
18. Weber, H. A contribution to the pathology of the crura cerebri. *Med. Chir. Trans* **1863**, *46*, 121–139. [CrossRef] [PubMed]
19. Benedikt, M. Tremblement avec paralysie croisée du mo- teur oculaire commun. *Bull. Med. Paris* **1889**, *3*, 547–548.
20. Wallenberg, A. Anatomischer Befund in einem als akute Bulbaraffection (Embolie der Arteria cerebelli inferior posterior sinistra) bescriebenen Falle. *Arch. Psychiatr.* **1901**, *34*, 923–959. [CrossRef]
21. Babinski, J.; Nageotte, J. Hémiasynergie, lateropulsion et myosis bulbaires avec hémianesthesie et hémiplegie croisees. *Rev. Neurol.* **1902**, *10*, 358–365.
22. Claude, H. Syndrome pedonculaire de la region du noyau rouge. *Rev. Neurol.* **1912**, *23*, 311–313.
23. Dejerine, J.; Roussy, G. Le syndrome thalamique. *Rev. Neurol.* **1906**, *14*, 521–532.
24. Foix, C.; Chavany, H.; Hillemand, P.; Schiff-Wertheimer, M. Obliteration del'artere choroïdienne anterieure: Ramollissement de son territoire cérébral: Hémiplégie, hémianesthésie et hémianopsie. *Bull. Soc. Ophtalmol. Fr.* **1925**, *27*, 221–223.
25. Foix, C.; Levy, M. Les ramollissements sylviens. *Rev. Neurol.* **1927**, *43*, 1–51.
26. Foix, C.; Hillemand, P. Les syndromes de l'artere cerebrale anterieure. *Encephale* **1925**, *20*, 209–232.
27. Foix, C.; Masson, A. Le syndrome de l'artere cerebrale posterieure. *Presse Med.* **1923**, *31*, 361–365.
28. Paciaroni, M.; Bogousslavsky, J. The history of stroke and cerebrovascular disease. *Handb. Clin. Neurol.* **2008**, *92*, 3–28.
29. Fields, W.S.; Lemak, N.A. *A History of Stroke*; Oxford University Press: New York, NY, USA, 1989.
30. Paciaroni, M.; Bogousslavsky, J. How did stroke become of interest to neurologists? A slow 19th century saga. *Neurology* **2009**, *73*, 724–728. [PubMed]

© 2023 by the authors. Licensee MDPI, Basel, Switzerland. This article is an open access article distributed under the terms and conditions of the Creative Commons Attribution (CC BY) license (http://creativecommons.org/licenses/by/4.0/).

Stroke and the Arts

Bartlomiej Piechowski-Jozwiak and Julien Bogousslavsky

Abstract: Stroke is the second leading cause of death, and it is a significant cause of disability on a global scale. The incidence and prevalence of stroke are rising, including in younger populations. Art can be seen as a means of universal communication, and artistic production can be seen as an ultimate achievement of the human brain. Visual art production requires multiple processes such as basic motor skills and more advanced associative functions such as visuospatial processing, emotional output, socio-cultural factoring and creativity. Focal and non-focal brain damage caused by stroke may lead to either the de novo occurrence of artistic productivity or a change in an established artistic style. In this chapter, we look at the historical development of the understanding of the role of stroke and stroke therapy in changing artistic output. We also discuss various examples of previously art-naïve individuals changing into prolific artists after stroke and established painters evolving new artistic styles after stroke.

1. Introduction

Stroke is the second leading cause of death, and it is a significant cause of disability on a global scale. The incidence and prevalence of stroke are rising, which is related to the aging of the general population and increasing incidence of stroke in younger populations [1]. The global lifetime risk of stroke increased from 1990 to 2016 from 22.8% to 24.9%, with the risk of ischemic stroke being higher (18.3%) than hemorrhagic stroke (8.2%). There are significant geographical, ethnic and economic differences in lifetime stroke risk, which is the highest in East Asian countries (38.8%), followed by Central Europe (31.7%) and Eastern Europe (31.6%), and the lowest in sub-Saharan Africa (11.8%) [2]. The burden of stroke can be seen from the perspective of long-term symptoms. Up to 37% of stroke survivors may experience a reduction in mobility, 45% of female and 39% of male patients may experience decreased handgrip and 29% may experience reduced dual-task capacity; in the cognitive domain, 33% may experience reduced global cognition, 37% may experience a degree of impairment of executive function and 39% may experience a reduction in memory [3]. Cognitive impairment without dementia before stroke increases the risk of post-stroke dementia within two years of follow-up [4]. Post-stroke cognitive impairment, including memory, language, orientation and attention deficits, increases functional disability and the odds of dependent living (unadjusted OR of 2.4) [5].

The impact of stroke on motor, behavioral and cognitive functions is substantial. The human brain is our evolutionary gain, and many brain functions, despite the significant advances in neuroscience, cannot at this stage be attributed solely to anatomical structures [6]. Interpersonal variabilities in intellectual abilities, empathy, compassion and creative skills provide a platform for variable capacity to produce, read and perceive art [6]. The role of art in conveying a universal message through expression and abstracting was assessed previously regarding the biological basis of this process and remote interactions between the artist and the art recipient [7]. Art can be seen as a dialogue platform between the expression of those interpersonal variabilities and the appreciation of the art product for its esthetic, emotional and intellectual meaning [7]. In this context, art serves as a timeless, supra-cultural and supra-religious connection between the artist and the art viewer [7]. The mechanisms underlying this unique interface are proposed to be based on symbolism with the exchange of unswerving and spontaneous expression between the artist and the viewer, reflecting a more profound biological information exchange related to survival and adaptation to the environment [7]. This information exchange was postulated to be related to the mirror neuron network interactions and frontoparietal bidirectional connections allowing for the sensory stimulus to trigger primary motor pathways [7].

The sensory attributes of the witnessed actions or emotions could activate the mirror neurons, triggering the motor depiction of the same activity within the observing brain [7]. The linking action of mirror neurons can connect perception and cognition as one domain. Hence, the first-person experience on the neuronal plane would be the same as the third-person experience, leading to a shared functional state [8]. The neurochemical pathways for artistic and creative activities were studied in healthy individuals challenged with divergent thinking tests that correlate positively with overall creativity. The subjects were assessed with positron emission tomography. The proposed transmitter was dopamine and its D2 receptor [9]. This study showed a negative relationship between divergent thinking and thalamic D2 receptor density, suggesting the importance of thalamic D2 receptors in creativity [9]. The decreased thalamic gating thresholds were suggested to play a role in increased thalamocortical information transfer, hence leading to increased creativity [9].

The complexity of artistic creation based on the involvement of multiple cortical areas and functioning white matter connections can be affected by focal damage caused by stroke. Most of the neurological deficits related to stroke leading to artistic changes are described in the context of focal symptoms of hemineglect, apraxia, perceptual agnosia, visual field deficits and focal damage in the regions of right-sided parietal and occipital areas, as well as dysphasia and left-hemispheric lesions [10]. These anatomic and clinical correlations of stroke involving the right cerebral hemisphere are linked to changes in spatial arrangements of the whole or part of a painting, and strokes confined to the left cerebral hemisphere are linked to abridgement of the painting details [10]. An exciting mechanism was observed in individuals with non-focal and stroke-unrelated conditions such as frontotemporal dementia, where predominantly left-hemispheric involvement would lead to decreased abilities to abstract, symbolize and enhance creative and emotional capacity [10,11]. In addition to the effects of a focal cortical function on art creation, one can also consider the networking within the brain and the role of interconnections of proximal and remote cortical areas in creative processes. The role of the brain connectome in creative thinking was studied recently with the use of functional MRI [12]. The main finding pertains to discovering centralized, hub-like brain cognitive structures linked by high-information traffic connections that allow for higher creative thinking [12]. The brain hubs related to the high creative potential were those providing sensorimotor, executive control and memory-based processing; this elevated creative potential was magnified by integration through the high-information traffic connections [12]. An interesting non-lateralized left-to-right model of a tripartite system consisting of temporal, frontal and limbic cortices in creativity in health and disease states was discussed previously [13]. The subtle interactions between those three hubs were proposed based on the temporal lobe driving idea generation with the frontal lobe's control and mesolimbic regions' influences on novelty seeking and creative drive through dopaminergic transmission [13]. These models and findings are essential in establishing a functional basis for the effects of different types of brain injury, including strokes, on artistic ability beyond just anatomical deficits and partial alteration of creative output.

The change in artistic style may involve altered artistic output in established artists or the development of "de novo" creative abilities in otherwise art-naïve individuals. Only a small number of individuals can express extraordinary artistic creativity using unorthodox and innovative techniques and methods; hence, the disease process affecting these capabilities and, consequently, altering artistic output provides a better understanding of the neurophysiology of the art [14]. The insights from the effects of focal neurological damage caused by a stroke on artistic creativity may help to understand the role of the brain connectome, cortical areas and neurochemical transmission in stroke recovery. This chapter assesses the impact of stroke on various types of art and artistic production in established artists and art-naïve individuals.

2. Change of Artistic Creativity in Established Artists

We start this journey with a historical perspective and the turn of the 19th and 20th centuries, when the attention of neurologists was drawn to changes observed in artists with neurological disorders including stroke [15]. One of the most historical artists with stroke was Lovis Corinth (1858–1925), whose artistic style was focused on the exact depiction of colors and the authenticity of naturalistic, mythological scenes, landscapes and still lives [16,17]. In 1911, he suffered from a sudden onset of left-sided weakness and ipsilateral lower homonymous quadrantanopia. He partially recovered from the stroke and could walk with support. His neurological diagnosis was established much later based on his symptoms and recovery [17]. He resumed painting after the stroke, and left-sided omissions, spatial deformities and zig-zag lines embedded in his painting were noted, which were consistent with hemineglect and hemifield pseudohallucinations [16,17].

In a larger historical cohort of 13 professional artists with right-hemispheric strokes, the authors observed significant changes in artistic output mostly related to emotional sequelae and negative neurological signs [18]. One of the earliest reported artists from this cohort was Anton Rädersheidt (1892–1970), who was known for starting the artistic trend in the mid-1920s known as "Magischer Realismus" (Magic Realism) discerned by photographic portrait details and a reduction in emotional content [18]. His artistic style evolved after 1950 into abstract expressionism. In 1967, he suffered from a stroke with mild left-sided weakness, severe left-sided homonymous hemianopia, left-sided hemineglect, spatial disorientation and severe prosopagnosia [18]. A few years after his stroke, Rädersheidt produced an extensive series of autoportraits that demonstrated the progressive improvement of his left-sided neglect, and his further paintings revealed a significant change in artistic style with an overload of vividly colorful strokes, depictions of ecstatic, sexually loaded scenes and picturing of disfigured bodies [18].

Another painter, Otto Dix (1891–1969), was recognized for his early naturalistic style with a focus on the everyday subject matter, including war scenes. The caricatural depiction of dreadful figures characterized his portraits, and critics considered his art as "degenerate" [18]. In 1967, he suffered from a stroke with left-sided weakness, left-arm dyspraxia with proprioceptive sensory impairment, hemianopia, hemineglect and spatial disturbance. In the initial phase post-stroke, Dix was unable to draw. With time, he overcame his hemineglect; his painting style changed, focusing on autoportraits with a decomposition of lines and painting structure, over-exaggeration of facial features and depictions of supernumerous fingers [18].

Reynold Brown (1917–1991) was a left-handed artist known for his initial engagement in illustrations of service manuals, pocketbooks, comics and magazines; he later started illustrating movie posters and record covers and eventually shifted to oil paintings of landscapes and portraits [18]. Brown suffered from a severe stroke in 1976 with profound left-sided weakness affecting his dominant arm, hemineglect and left lower quadrantanopia. After a period of intensive recovery supported by his family, he started painting, and the immediate change in his style was the marginalization of the left lower side of the canvas related to his quadrantanopia, stretching the content from the top right to the lower left, but also a distortion of facial features [18]. Notably, Brown's new artistic style carried a more emotional load than his initial realistic works by loosening the landscapes and using more colors [18].

Tom Greenshields (1915–1994) was a proficient sculptor and painter who had a dominant right-arm injury a few years prior to the onset of a stroke, which made him shift to using his left arm for artistic production [18]. In 1989, he suffered from a stroke with mild left-sided weakness, sensory impairment, hemineglect and lower quadrantanopia, and despite regaining left-arm function, his artistic output changed significantly with decreased structure, less extravagant drawings and an apparent impact of his neglect, with distortions, deformations, missing details and exaggeration of the figures on the left side [18].

Overall, this series of artists with right-hemispheric strokes shows a pattern in changing artistic output mainly related to emotional and mood stroke sequelae and negative neurological signs, including visual defects, hemineglect, prosopagnosia and spatial perception disturbances.

The role of hemineglect in the change in drawing style is clearly depicted in Federico Fellini's (1920–1993) recovery after a stroke. Fellini is known as a prolific film director, winning multiple international awards, but less is known about his initial career as a journalist, playwright, cartoonist and caricaturist working for the comic magazine *Marc Aurelio* and drawing caricatures of American marines [19]. At 73, he suffered from an ischemic stroke in the posterior right middle cerebral artery territory with severe left-sided hemiparesis, sensory loss, left inferior quadrantanopia and severe ipsilateral visuospatial hemineglect and misoplegia (negative perception of the paretic limbs) [19]. In his post-stroke sketching, he showed clear signs of visual and spatial neglect by omitting and simplifying the left side of the drawings and completing them later, which was a sign of him being aware of his visual and spatial neglect (Figure 1) [19].

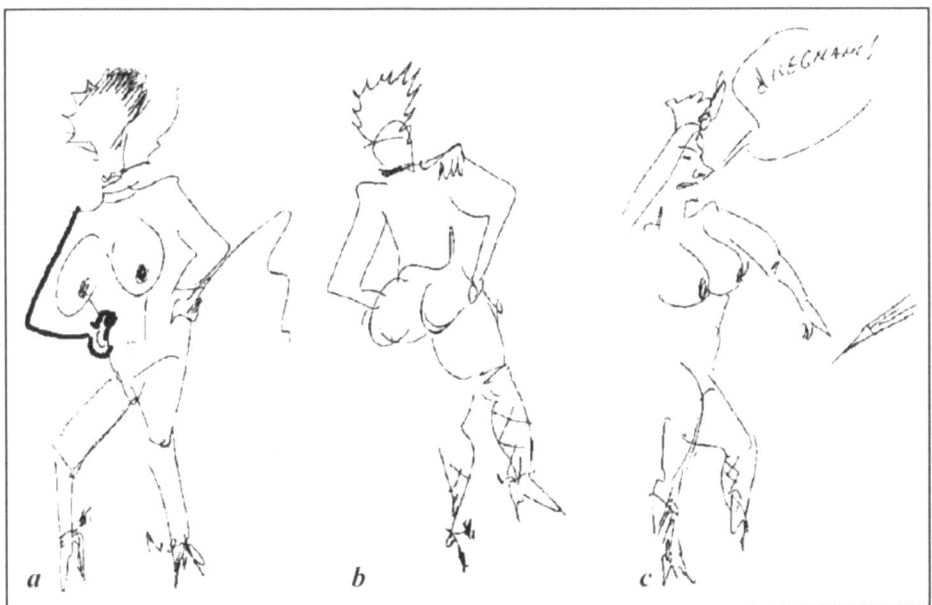

Figure 1. Fellini's drawing 25 days post-stroke of a female from different perspectives (front (**a**), back (**b**), profile (**c**)). Of note is the missing part of the drawings on the left side. In drawing (**a**), Fellini realized his left-sided deficiency and added a drawing of the right arm with a different pen. In drawing (**c**), he added the text "draw me!" (Source: Reprinted from Cantagallo and Della Sala, 1998, with permission) [20].

He recovered from his left-sided neglect within two months, and it is essential to note that he suffered from extrapersonal neglect, which he was aware of. After a few weeks following his stroke, his drawings revealed a complete perception of the sensorium and the disappearance of his neglect [19].

Another example is the case of Boris Krasnov (1961–2021), who was a world-known stage designer, prolific artistic producer, screenwrighter, sculptor and painter [21]. Krasnov had a right middle cerebral artery infarction complicated by left-sided weakness and significant hemineglect. He drew a portrait sketch of his treating physician a few months after his stroke that clearly demonstrated left-sided neglect (Figure 2).

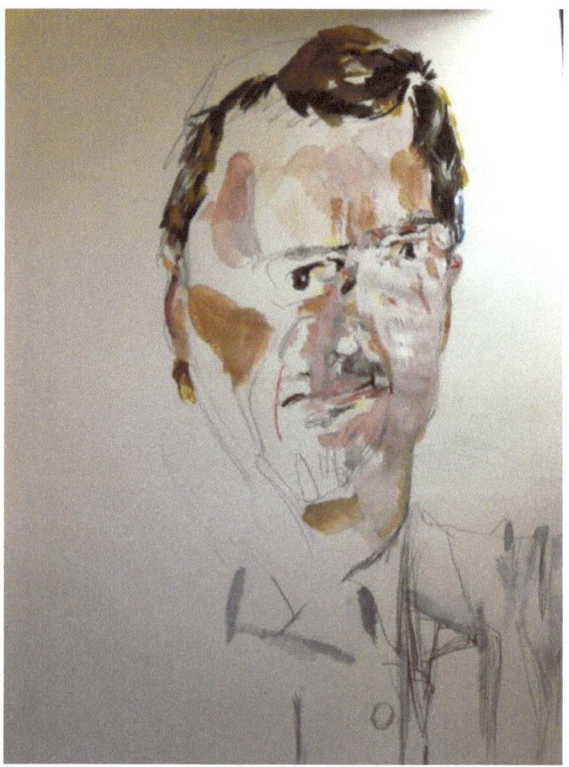

Figure 2. Credit: © Boris Krasnov's portrait sketch of Prof. Julien Bogousslavsky (used with permission).

A further example of a 20th century artist is an ambidextrous female Polish painter and sculptor, Krystyna Habura, who was born in 1928 and died in 1994 [22]. She was an established artist, receiving multiple international awards and exhibiting her works in Poland and internationally; she was known for her expressive paintings using rich colors, abstractionism, figurative painting and relentless experimentation with her style and techniques [22]. She focused on portraits ranging from realistic depictions to surrealistic symbolism (Figure 3).

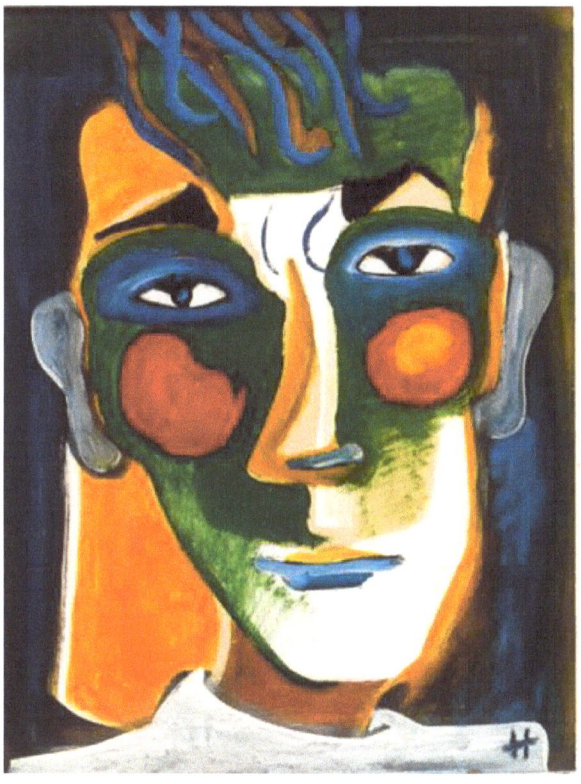

Figure 3. Krystyna Habura pre-stroke painting (Elfik) (Credit: © Pachalska M., used with permission [22]).

Her artistic production was dynamic and came in intense waves of creativity, with days or weeks spent on painting, alcohol use, smoking, and poor sleep and food hygiene [22]. Together with her cardiovascular risks (hypertension), these creative spells led to an ischemic stroke in the right middle cerebral artery territory with left-sided weakness, Luria's dynamic aphasia and spatial orientation dysfunction [22]. Following her stroke, she needed multiple inpatient rehabilitation programs where she re-learnt to walk and improved her speech, dexterity and ability to deal with activities of daily living [22]. The most disturbing symptom remaining after the stroke was, as defined by Habura, "creative aphasia", with the inability to paint and missing the drive she had previously to create [22]. During her expertly guided art therapy sessions, she started with right-hand sketching and then moved to support her left-hand movements with the right hand, allowing for the left hand to regain sufficient dexterity for independent drawing and painting [22]. After extended multistage therapy, her artistic creativity returned with changes in her style to a more sketch-like, simplified and logically detached pattern (Figure 4) [23].

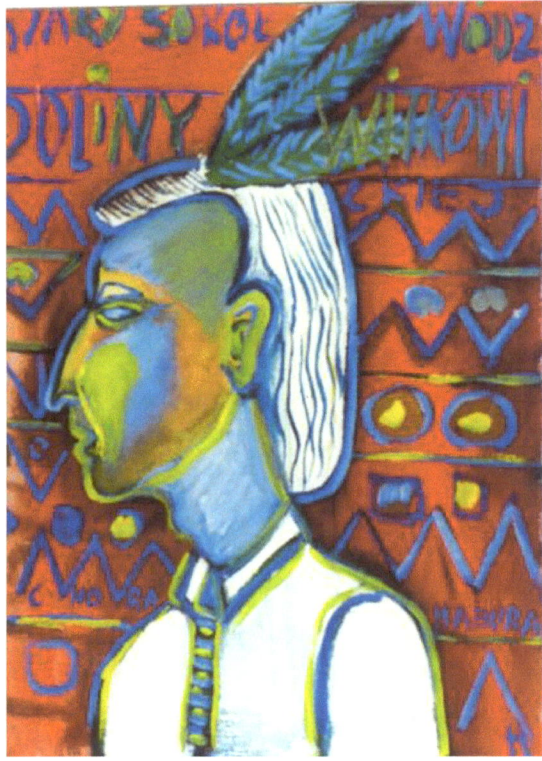

Figure 4. Habura's post-stroke painting "Grey Hawk, Chief of the Witkowice Tribe" (Credit: © Pachalska M., used with permission).

It is interesting to see opposite changes in the two individuals developing de novo artistic creativity and the established artist becoming unable to create at the previous momentum despite her neurological recovery of focal deficits. The previously mentioned interactions between the temporal and frontal cortices and idea and artistic drive control can explain some of these opposing developments in artistic creation.

Non-focal neurological deficits were shown to alter the artistic output in individuals with posterior circulation strokes. Annoni et al. [10] reported on a 57-year-old self-taught right-handed lithographer whose painting was focused on simplified figurative themes and geometric shapes and used a naïve and expressive style [10]. He presented with sudden-onset right superior quadrantanopia, with sparing of macular vision, difficulties with identifying complex objects in the upper right visual field and autoscopia—he saw his own body on the floor with his head turned to the left. Magnetic resonance imaging (MRI) confirmed an infarction within the visual cortex involving the primary and secondary sensory areas; his ancillary tests did not reveal the underlying etiology, and he was diagnosed with cryptogenic stroke [10]. During his recovery, the quadrantanopia evolved into recurrent photopsias and dyschromatopsia in the previously affected visual field with a corresponding paracentral scotoma [10]. A long-term follow-up assessment revealed delays in visual detection tasks, veering off a discourse topic consistent with a dysexecutive syndrome, and elements of post-traumatic stress disorder (PTSD), but his overall functioning and activities of daily living returned to normal [10]. After resuming his artistic activity, changes were noted, such as simplification of details, painting thinner and more stylized extremities and the use of simplified colors; he also started inserting glowing shapes in the area of his persistent scotoma [10]. He also noticed changes in his inspiration, with it coming immediately prior to painting, but previous to his stroke, he would contemplate the production for a while ahead [10].

The second case is a 71-year-old ambidextrous artist who started his career after the age of 50 and gained a local and national reputation by producing figurative and impressionist paintings of Swiss landscapes [10]. He suffered from a left paramedian thalamic infarction and resolving symptoms of right-sided ataxia, hypoesthesia and weakness; the stroke etiology was cardioembolic (atrial fibrillation) [10]. In a long-term follow-up assessment, he was found to have mild to moderate dysexecutive symptoms with verbal and figural perseverations and decreased precision in imaginary tasks [10]. He regained the ability to paint a few weeks after the stroke and started using both hands interchangeably despite regaining full dexterity of the dominant right hand. His clients and art critics noted this a few months after, and he moved from a figurative style to a more detail-focused, spatially structured and color-realistic style; the artist himself commented on the change as becoming more sensitive to natural beauty and expressing the rawness of it in his paintings, shifting away from impressionism as it lacked the realism [10]. His left hand allowed him to discover stronger colors, express emotions better and become more creative [10].

The overlapping theme in both of these artists is a change in artistic drive, attention to detail and the use of colors. These transformations went in the opposite directions: the first artist turned to simplicity in colors and details, with an alteration in artistic drive; the other turned to more complex spatial arrangements, increased attention to detail and vivid colors, with increased artistic creativity. The artistic changes observed in these two artists are, in part, related to the dysexecutive syndrome. There was no correlation between the localization of the stroke and defined or reproducible changes in painting style.

The following report brings a greater understanding of the changes in artistic style after a posterior circulation stroke. An 87-year-old established artist presented with sudden-onset vertigo, horizontal diplopia with partial left oculomotor nerve palsy, dysarthria, right facial droop, right-arm weakness, and gait and truncal ataxia consistent with posterior circulation ischemic stroke; computed tomography of her brain showed previous symmetrical small vessel changes in the basal ganglia [24]. Her condition improved after her stroke, with resolution of gait ataxia and right-arm weakness and persistence of subjective diplopia despite the normal neuro-ophthalmological evaluation; upon neuropsychological assessment, she was found to have significant constructional apraxia and attention deficit [24]. She resumed painting within four weeks of the stroke. Her premorbid paintings were dedicated to architectural objects and flowers, and all were painted from visual memory and modified before putting them on canvas [24]. The premorbid and two-year post-stroke paintings showed her ability to paint the whole image and center the object of interest accordingly. Her paintings developed during her stroke recovery; of note, however, is the fact that she did not remember painting any of these, showed a selective focus on parts of the work and was unable to develop the whole of the object, which was attributed to problems with simultaneous creativity and storage of visual memory [24]. In this artist, the unique combination of visual memory translation in her painting with the inability to translate the wholeness of her imagination and a selective focus on parts of the visual creation is suggestive of visual agnosia and asimultagnosia, possibly linked to dysfunction of the associative visual cortex function with an aberrant abstraction of visual input and interpretation of visual memories [24].

Another insight into artistic creativity and stroke comes from the case of Carl Frederik Reutersward (1934–2016), a right-handed multilingual (he was able to speak Swedish as a primary language, and English, French and German as secondary languages) sculptor and painter who suffered from an intracerebral hemorrhage within the left-sided lenticular nucleus and internal capsule, which caused right-sided weakness, sensory loss and subcortical aphasia affecting all four languages, with Swedish being least affected [25]. In a long-term follow-up assessment, he was found to have ongoing right-arm weakness, moderate dysexecutive syndrome, minimal visual agnosia and resolution of his dysphasia [25]. He attempted painting with the paralyzed right arm to stimulate recovery, but after a long period of intense rehab, he later started using his non-dominant hand, which he found beneficial to his artistic creativity. He described his new gift with the following words:

> "... it's marvellous... it's not a handicap... the left hand is the dreamer... the soul is localized in the left hand" [25]

Following the change of creative side to the left arm, his artistic output changed, with a greater emotional load and artistic intensity. Art critics noted this and praised him for gaining expressiveness, freshness, vitality, psychic intensity and playfulness [25]. A great example is his premorbid sketch of a pistol ("Non-Violence"), which was drawn with hefty and decisive strokes. After his stroke, he drew the lethal pistol again, but the drawing was humoristic and pictured the weapon as a toy [25].

There is a parallel between the changes observed in Reutersward's style and the second case of posterior circulation stroke, as both artists switched from the right dominant to the left non-dominant hand. Both observed greater expressiveness, emotional load and creativity, but there were opposite shifts to playfulness and humor in the former and realism in the latter.

3. De Novo Artistic Creativity in Brain Disorders

A fascinating insight comes from more contemporary examples of individuals developing a sudden artistic output due to cerebrovascular disease with predominantly non-focal cerebral involvement, emphasizing the role of networks and intercortical communication in artistic output. The first example is of a 35-year-old chiropractor, Mr Jon Sarkin (born in 1953), who in 1988 suffered from a left cerebellar hemorrhage and hypoxic brain injury caused by two heart arrests after an elective neurosurgical procedure for correcting a neurovascular conflict at the level of the acoustic nerve; he required decompressive surgery and partial cerebellar parenchyma removal [26,27]. Following his stroke, he remained in a coma, and during his recovery, he transformed from a quiet and reserved person into an unpredictable, uncontrollable, unconventional, creative artist. Part of his change was related to cognitive symptoms related to his hypoxic episode and impairment of fresh memory [27]. He did not have any formal artistic formation, but he had the drive to produce surreal and complicated artworks [28]. He commented on his transformation with the following words:

I do think it (art) was always latent inside me... But I did not suddenly feel motivated after my stroke. It was just what I did and do. It's a bit like asking you if you feel motivated to breathe? You just do it. It was an autonomic thing. [28]

Sarkin started his drawings initially with random doodling with curves, zig-zags and spiral lines portraying old cars, animals or plants. His artistic style progressed and became more advanced, and he was noticed as an artist after sending his work to the *New Yorker* magazine [28]. This sudden and constant burst of creativity transformed his life entirely. His artistic production took over all his previous activities and made him paint, draw, write poems and imbed words into his art [27] (Figure 5).

Sarkin described the urge for creation and the relation between his stroke and the drive to produce art in the following words:

"[My artwork is] a manifestation of what happened to me... I've learned how to visually represent my existential dilemma caused by my stroke." [29]

He became a very prolific artist, exhibiting his works in the best venues. Sarkin's transformation and journey through his disease and related disability, or rather new ability, are an excellent reflection of the human potential to recover and the brain's potential to regenerate and, despite ongoing cognitive symptoms, expand into new means of communication [27] (Figure 6).

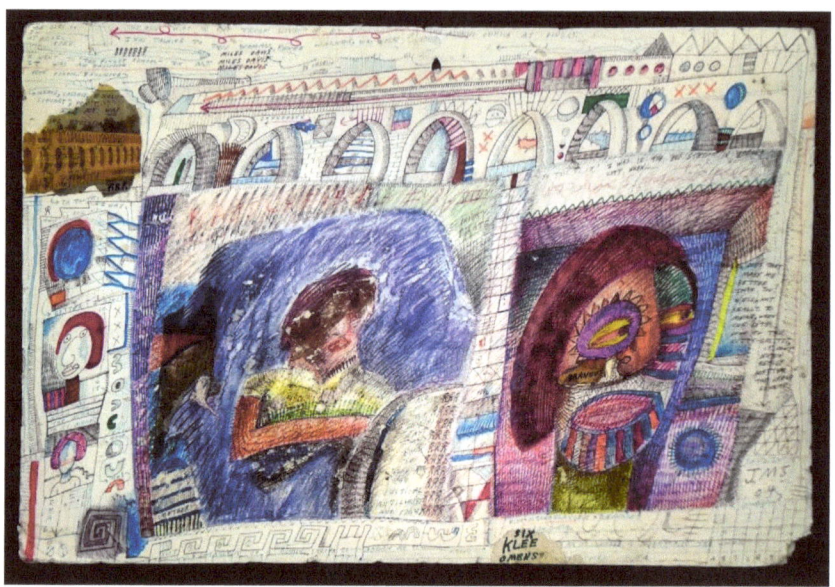

Figure 5. Sarkin's painting (Image 202_10925_135520_292_HDR-01), Credit: © Sarkin J., used with permission.

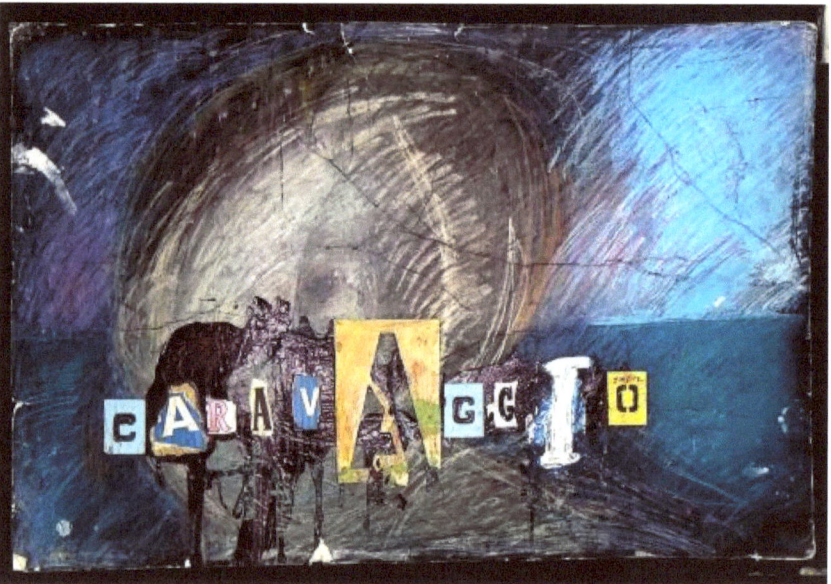

Figure 6. Sarkin's painting (IMG_20-210925_134719594_HDR-01), Credit: © Sarkin J., used with permission.

There is another example of a sudden artistic output in a stroke survivor. This is the case of Tommy McHugh (1949–2012), who suffered from non-focal brain damage caused by a subarachnoid hemorrhage [30]. After his hemorrhage, he required aneurysmal coiling and clipping, and he remained comatose for ten days. McHugh did not have any formal artistic training, and prior to the onset of his hemorrhage, he worked as a builder; in his youth, he served his time in prison, and he had a long history of substance abuse [30]. He described the sudden change leading to artistic production with the following words:

> *I suddenly felt an explosion in the left side of my head and ended up on the floor... . Then the other side of my head went bang! I woke up in hospital and looked out of the window to see the tree was sprouting numbers. 3, 6, 9. Then I started talking in rhyme...* [30]

With his creative compulsions for poetry and pictorial activity, McHugh made the following remarkable statement:

> *I just plough into it, finish it, move away and then go and maybe make a clay head. I finish that and go and play with a bit of stone, come back and do another picture, sit down and write a poem, get up and make a butterfly out of birds' feathers.* [31]

He volunteered to be examined by prominent neurologists, and based on his neuropsychological assessment, he was diagnosed with frontal lobe dysfunction with verbal disinhibition and impaired multitasking [30]. He described his outpour of creative impulses with the following words:

> "*It's like Mount Etna exploding. Fairy liquid bubbles of intelligence and they are popping around me all the time—grabbing one and trying to remember it before it floats away, popping.*" [30]

The uninhibited drive to create made him paint on the walls, ceilings and floors; in addition to this, he noticed changes in his personality, with excessive emotionality, and discovered the feminine aspects of his nature [30]. His poetry also showed references to the overflow of contextual expression in any available space and the endless need to find the meaning of the blindfolded creation ("I am climbing the mountains...") [32].

These examples of de novo artistic creativity show some similarities with stroke-related non-focal brain injury and more diffuse changes in the functional connectivity and brain function with the overflow of pictorial and verbal expressions that were transformed into art pieces. The lack of laterality in the brain injuries in these two cases sheds new light on the artistic changes related to stroke with de novo creativity. In addition, one may postulate the role of temporal and frontal cortical connections, with a relative switch in the balance to releasing idea generation from the temporal areas with less frontal inhibition.

Art therapy was mentioned above in the case studies of artists affected by stroke to improve stroke-related symptoms. Art therapy was discovered and named for the first time by Adrian Hill in 1942, who was recovering from tuberculosis; he discovered the therapeutic benefits of visual arts, such as the release of creative energy and resilience building. In addition to this, he recommended art therapy to his peer patients [33]. Creative-art-based therapies focus on specific types of artistic output, including music, dance and visual arts such as painting and drawing. The diverse forms of therapy focus on various functions and deficit dipoles. However, the common goal is to deliver multisource stimulation and boost creativity to allow for functional restoration, psychological support, social engagement and spiritual experiences [34]. Visual-art-based therapies were shown to increase self-expression, enhance confidence and mood and allow for relaxation, distraction, encouragement and a sense of control [34]. In the case of visual art therapy, more focal deficits such as spatial awareness and extremity weakness are targeted, which may improve functional outcomes [35].

4. Summary

Art can be considered as a means of universal communication that is timeless and not limited by cultural constraints, and art production can be seen as an ultimate achievement of the human brain. Historical observations from established artists whose productivity was altered by stroke allow us to understand two patterns. The first includes loss of function that degrades the organization of the painting plane, omitting and neglecting a part of it or including representations of visual field defects as part of the production. The second pattern involves a loss of or change in artistic drive, with the spectrum ranging from "artistic aphasia" to mechanical creation, and alteration of the emotional content, from overload to complete dryness and distancing. The occurrence of de novo artistic skills in otherwise art-naïve individuals shows the great potential that sits in all of us. The trigger of the nascent artistic productivity discussed in this paper is related to focal and non-focal brain injuries, and increases in artistic drive can be attributed to the change in the balance of interactions among different cortical regions in the frontal–posterior relation rather than disruption of right- or left-sided function. The language of art and artistic production can both be used in helping stroke survivors recover through art therapy. They can also help to establish a non-verbal communication portal bypassing neurological disease.

Author Contributions: Conceptualization, B.P.-J. and J.B.; methodology, B.P.-J., J.B.; writing—original draft preparation, B.P.-J.; writing—review and editing, J.B.; visualization, B.P.-J., J.B. All authors have read and agreed to the published version of the manuscript.

Funding: This research received no external funding.

Conflicts of Interest: The authors declare no conflict of interest.

References

1. Katan, M.; Luft, A. Global Burden of Stroke. *Semin. Neurol.* **2018**, *38*, 208–211. [CrossRef]
2. The GBD 2016 Lifetime Risk of Stroke Collaborators. Global, Regional, and Country-Specific Lifetime Risks of Stroke, 1990 and 2016. *N. Engl. J. Med.* **2018**, *379*, 2429–2437. [CrossRef]

3. Einstad, M.S.; Saltvedt, I.; Lydersen, S.; Ursin, M.H.; Munthe-Kaas, R.; Ihle-Hansen, H.; Knapskog, A.-B.; Askim, T.; Beyer, M.K.; Næss, H.; et al. Associations between Post-Stroke Motor and Cognitive Function: A Cross-Sectional Study. *BMC Geriatr.* **2021**, *21*, 103. [CrossRef]
4. Serrano, S.; Domingo, J.; Rodríguez-Garcia, E.; Castro, M.-D.; del Ser, T. Frequency of Cognitive Impairment Without Dementia in Patients With Stroke. *Stroke* **2007**, *38*, 105–110. [CrossRef]
5. Tatemichi, T.K.; Desmond, D.W.; Stern, Y.; Paik, M.; Sano, M.; Bagiella, E. Cognitive Impairment after Stroke: Frequency, Patterns, and Relationship to Functional Abilities. *J. Neurol. Neurosurg. Psychiatry* **1994**, *57*, 202–207. [CrossRef]
6. Zeki, S. Essays on Science and Society. Artistic Creativity and the Brain. *Science* **2001**, *293*, 51–52. [CrossRef]
7. Piechowski-Jozwiak, B.; Boller, F.; Bogousslavsky, J. Universal Connection through Art: Role of Mirror Neurons in Art Production and Reception. *Behav. Sci.* **2017**, *7*, 29. [CrossRef]
8. Gallese, V. Mirror Neurons and Art. In *Art and the Senses*; Oxford University Press: Oxford, UK, 2013; pp. 441–449.
9. de Manzano, Ö.; Cervenka, S.; Karabanov, A.; Farde, L.; Ullén, F. Thinking Outside a Less Intact Box: Thalamic Dopamine D2 Receptor Densities Are Negatively Related to Psychometric Creativity in Healthy Individuals. *PLoS ONE* **2010**, *5*, e10670. [CrossRef]
10. Annoni, J.; Devuyst, G.; Carota, A.; Bruggimann, L.; Bogousslavsky, J. Changes in Artistic Style after Minor Posterior Stroke. *J. Neurol. Neurosurg. Psychiatry* **2005**, *76*, 797. [CrossRef]
11. Piechowski-Jozwiak, B.; Bogousslavsky, J. Abstract Expressionists and Brain Disease. In *Neurological Disorders in Famous Artists—Part 4*; Bogousslavsky, J., Tatu, L., Eds.; Karger: Berlin, Germany, 2018; pp. 8–22. [CrossRef]
12. Zhuang, K.; Yang, W.; Li, Y.; Zhang, J.; Chen, Q.; Meng, J.; Wei, D.; Sun, J.; He, L.; Mao, Y.; et al. Connectome-Based Evidence for Creative Thinking as an Emergent Property of Ordinary Cognitive Operations. *Neuroimage* **2021**, *227*, 117632. [CrossRef]
13. Flaherty, A.W. Frontotemporal and Dopaminergic Control of Idea Generation and Creative Drive. *J. Comp. Neurol.* **2005**, *493*, 147–153. [CrossRef] [PubMed]
14. Bogousslavsky, J.; Boller, F.; Hennerici, M.G. *Neurological Disorders in Famous Artists*; Part 2; Bogousslavsky, J., Hennerici, M.G., Eds.; Karger: Berlin, Germany, 2007.
15. Jung, R. Neuropsychologie Und Neurophysiologie Des Kontur-Und Formsehens in Zeichnung Und Malerei. In *Psychopathologie Musischer Gestaltungen*; Wieck, H.H., Ed.; Schattauer: Erlangen, Germany, 1974; pp. 29–88.
16. Blanke, O. VisuoSpatial Neglect In Lovis Corinth's Self-Portraits. *Int. Rev. Neurobiol.* **2006**, *74*, 193–214. [CrossRef] [PubMed]
17. Blanke, O.; Pasqualini, I. The Riddle of Style Changes in the Visual Arts after Interference with the Right Brain. *Front. Hum. Neurosci.* **2012**, *5*, 154. [CrossRef] [PubMed]
18. Bäzner, H.; Hennerici, M.G. Painting after Right-Hemisphere Stroke—Case Studies of Professional Artists. *Front. Neurol. Neurosci.* **2007**, *22*, 1–13. [CrossRef] [PubMed]
19. Dieguez, S.; Assal, G.; Bogousslavsky, J. Visconti and Fellini: From Left Social Neorealism to Right-Hemisphere Stroke. *Front. Neurol. Neurosci.* **2007**, *22*, 44–74. [CrossRef] [PubMed]

20. Cantagallo, A.; Sala, S.D. Preserved Insight in an Artist with Extrapersonal Spatial Neglect. *Cortex* **1998**, *34*, 163–189. [CrossRef]
21. Zayakin, A. Died Screenwriter Pugacheva Boris Krasnov. *World Today News*, 2021. Available online: https://www.world-today-news.com/died-screenwriter-pugacheva-boris-krasnov/ (accessed on 18 May 2023).
22. Pąchalska, M.; Grochmal-Bach, B.; Wilk, M.; Buliński, L. Rehabilitation of an Artist after Right-Hemisphere Stroke. *Med. Sci. Monit.* **2008**, *14*, CS110-24.
23. Piechowski-Jozwiak, B.; Bogousslavsky, J. Painting in Neurology. *Brain Art* **2020**, 41–52. [CrossRef]
24. Smith, W.S.; Mindelzun, R.E.; Miller, B. Simultanagnosia through the Eyes of an Artist. *Neurology* **2003**, *60*, 1832–1834. [CrossRef]
25. Colombo-Thuillard, F.; Assal, G. Persisting Aphasia, Cerebral Dominance, and Painting in the Famous Artist Carl Fredrik Reuterswärd. *Front. Neurol. Neurosci.* **2007**, *22*, 169–183. [CrossRef]
26. Edgers, G. A Changed Man. 2006. Available online: http://archive.boston.com/ae/theater_arts/articles/2006/06/11/a_changed_man// (accessed on 18 May 2023).
27. Nutt, A.E. *Shadows Bright as Glass: The Remarkable Story of One Man's Journey from Brain Trauma to Artistic Triumph*; Free Press PP: New York, NY, USA, 2011.
28. Spencer, K. My Stroke Turned Me into an Artist. 2011. Available online: https://www.express.co.uk/ (accessed on 31 March 2022).
29. Gross, T. Jon Sarkin: When Brain Injuries Transform into Art. *90.5 WESA*, 2011. Available online: https://www.wesa.fm/2011-04-18/jon-sarkin-when-brain-injuries-transform-into-art (accessed on 31 March 2022).
30. Thomson, H. Mindscapes: Stroke Turned Ex-Con into Rhyming Painter. *New Scientist*. 2013. Available online: https://www.newscientist.com/article/dn23523-mindscapes-stroke-turned-ex-con-into-rhyming-painter/ (accessed on 31 March 2022).
31. Creative Side Unlocked by Stroke. 2004. Available online: https://www.news.bbc.co.uk (accessed on 31 March 2022).
32. McHugh, T. Poetry—Tommy McHugh. 2022. Available online: www.tommymchugh.co.uk (accessed on 31 March 2022).
33. Hogan, S. Healing Arts: The History of Art Therapy. *Heal. Arts Hist. Art Ther.* **2001**, *53*, 135.
34. Ting Lo, T.L.; Lee, J.L.C.; Ho, R.T.H. Creative Arts-Based Therapies for Stroke Survivors: A Qualitative Systematic Review. *Front. Psychol.* **2018**, *9*, 1646. [CrossRef]
35. Reynolds, F. Art Therapy after Stroke: Evidence and a Need for Further Research. *Arts Psychother.* **2012**, *39*, 239–244. [CrossRef]

© 2023 by the authors. Licensee MDPI, Basel, Switzerland. This article is an open access article distributed under the terms and conditions of the Creative Commons Attribution (CC BY) license (http://creativecommons.org/licenses/by/4.0/).

Part II: The 20th Century Revolution

The Interest in the Pathology and Pathophysiology of Vascular Lesions

Giorgio Silvestrelli

Abstract: This chapter presents the historical and progressive interest in cerebrovascular lesions which began in the 17th century. Despite its frequent occurrence, knowledge of the natural history of cerebrovascular disease was surprisingly scanty until 18th century. The history of cerebrovascular lesions covers several centuries, although the observations influencing current practice have been analyzed only since the 20th century. This chapter is a review of the contributions of the principal physicians, pathologists, anatomists, anthropologists, philosophers, pathoanatomists, neuropathologists and neurologists to the present knowledge of the pathology and pathophysiology of cerebrovascular lesions. The period from the 16th to the 20th century has been analyzed; the pathophysiology of cerebrovascular lesions has been divided according to etiological classification. The greatest contributions to knowledge are due to Felix Platter (1536–1614), Johann Jakob Wepfer (1620–1695), Giovanni Battista Morgagni (1682–1771), Jean André Rochoux (1787–1852), Léon Rostan (1790–1866), Karl von Rokitansky (1804–1878), Charles Louis Maxime Durand-Fardel (1815–1899), Rudolf Ludwig Virchow (1821–1902), Jean-Martin Charcot (1825–1893), Joseph Jules Déjerine (1849–1917), Pierre Marie (1853–1940), Charles Foix (1882–1927), Charles Miller-Fisher (1913–2012). At the end of the 19th century, the development of clinical–anatomic correlation studies of cerebrovascular lesions was considered a brain condition worthy of specific research and future knowledge.

1. Introduction

Progressive interest in the pathology and pathophysiology of cerebrovascular lesions (CVLs) began in the 17th and 18th centuries, mainly through autopsy findings, though cerebrovascular disease (CVD) remained unknown to many physicians in the 18th century.

The development of knowledge of CVD, was sluggish until the first half of the 19th century when the vascular nature of CVD was widely identified and accepted [1,2]. With the beginning of the 19th, CVD was defined for the first time as a result of a CVL (ischemic or/and hemorrhagic).

Morphological lesions alone defined the decisive criterion to indicate a CVD; the symptoms were then considered solely as "indicatory signs" and "pathological anatomy" established the key basis for all CVD knowledge [3]. The 20th century represented a revolution in CVL knowledge.

Interest in CVLs among pathologists, anthropologists, philosophers, physicians, neuropathologists, and neurologists was promoted by the development of clinical–topographical correlation studies carried out by Joseph Jules Déjerine

(1849–1917) and Pierre Marie (1853–1940), followed by Charles Foix (1882–1927), the forerunner of modern clinical CVD research.

2. History of Cerebrovascular Lesions

The first mention to the nervous system is discovered in the Edwin Smith Surgical Papyrus dating from 3500 BC, with the first reference to "brain" [4].

A sound knowledge of ancient doctrines regarding health and disease is necessary to comprehend Greco-Roman medical texts dealing with CVD.

In the Middle Ages, from 500 AD to 1500, the focus was on miraculous healing and the concept of medicine was aligned with religious practices thus not creating much scientific interest. This could justify why anatomopathological awareness of CVLs lagged so far behind morphological anatomy.

In the 14th century, the first anatomical analyses of human bodies were carried out; in the middle of the 15th century, larger numbers of post-mortem examination were executed, resulting in improved knowledge of brain anatomy and cerebral vessels.

Subsequently, in the 16th century, through the verification of the first autopsies it was possible to document the anatomical lesions linked to some diseases. This marked the birth of pathological anatomy [2].

2.1. CVL History in the 17th Century

In 1602, following the death of one of his CVD patients, Felix Platter (1536–1614), performed a brain autopsy. He summarized his findings in this way "a phlegmatic humour is obstructing the inner passages of the brain" [5].

This sentence allows us to highlight two fundamental aspects of the historical study of diseases: (i) in the past as in the present, every scientific observation is theory-based; (ii) clearly it is extremely difficult to counteract traditional beliefs. Platter had supported Galen's belief that phlegm in the cerebral ventricles caused apoplexy, and indeed the brain post-mortem confirmed the presence of phlegm in the cerebral cavities.

Johann Jakob Wepfer (1620–1695), one of the most renowned authors of his time, wrote numerous medical monographs during the 17th century in which CVD was defined only as a set of various symptoms. He made an accurate description of the anatomy of cerebral vessels with anterior arterial, many years before Willis. He was one of the first physician to compare the neurological manifestations with the results of the brain autopsy and hypothesized a possible correlation, thus paving the way for the subsequent anatomo-clinical method.

In the 17th century, accurate descriptions of the cerebral vessels and the first detailed analyses of the consequences of occlusion began to appear.

The humoral theory met its end in 1628 when William Harvey (1578–1657) described vascular circulation in the treatise "Exercitatio anatomica de motu cordis et sanguinis in animalibus" or, as it came to be known, "De motu cordis". He was intrigued by humoral circulation in the human body. At that time, it was widely believed that the liver converted food into blood which the body employed as fuel.

Up until the 1600s, it was thought that there were two distinct blood systems in the body. In the former, purple (nutritional) blood circulated through the veins to distribute nourishment from the liver to the rest of the body. In the second, scarlet (life-giving or vital) blood circulated through the arteries to deliver a life-giving principle from the lungs. At that time, the presence of oxygen in the blood was not known and it was thought that the circulation of the blood occurred around the body and consumed as it was produced. Circulation through the capillaries, small arteries and veins were unknown at the time and their presence was only discovered thanks to the microscope at the end of the 17th century.

By comparing clinical features with autopsy, Giovanni Battista Morgagni (1682–1771), an Italian anatomist, laid the foundations of clinical anatomic studies in CVD [6]. He promoted the anatomo-clinical approach in medicine which thus became the anatomical means to identify the origin and etiology of any disease. He also maintained the ancient apoplexy classification between "sanguineous" (hemorrhagic) vs. "serous" (no hemorrhagic) [7]. Furthermore, he subdivided hemorrhagic lesion in blood CVL (intracerebral hemorrhage) and water CVL (bleeding into the right ventricle) through the dissection of the brain analyzed.

2.2. CVL History in the 18th Century

Between the 17th and 18th centuries, evolving concepts of brain "softening" and "apoplexia" were consolidated [2]. Jean André Rochoux (1787–1852) claimed in 1814 that apoplexy was always the result of bleeding [8]. Apoplexy was described as "a sudden but mostly general, rather than focal, disorder of the brain".

In the period from 1820 to 1823, "spontaneous cerebral softening" is a different find from encephalitis and apoplexy was first defined by Léon Luis Rostan (1790–1866), a French pathologist, physicist and a representative of the anatomico-clinical School of Paris. The main finding of Rostan reported in his studies regarding CVD was his definition of "cerebral softening" (encephalomalacia), fundamental in the knowledge of CVLs. He no longer used CVD as a general term, regarding it as synonymous with hemorrhagic CVL.

He reported pathologic and clinical features of brain softening, which differed from apoplexy. In contrast to apoplexy, from which he had seen recovery, he declared softening to be fatal. He equated it with senile gangrene and retained that it was related to the "ossification" of cerebral arteries.

2.3. CVL History in the 19th Century

The definition of brain "softening" was opposed by authors such as François Joseph Victor Broussais (1772–1832) (from Lallemand, 1830 to Calmeil, 1859), who considered the brain softenings such as the result of "inflammation", hence the name encephalitis.

Conversely, Léon Rostan's proposals were accepted and elaborated by the Englishman Carswell (1835), the Scot Abercrombie (1836), and the Frenchman Andral (1827, 1840). While Léon Rostan had underlined a connection between an arterial condition (ossification) and parenchymatous lesions in his "Recherches sur les ramollissements du cerveau" (1823) he did not associate them with vessel blockage.

In 1856, this new concept was refused until the description of thromboembolism by the German Rudolf Ludwig Virchow (1821–1902), pathologist, statesman and anthropologist [2–9], and the studies of Adrien Proust (1862), Vincent Laborde (1866), Jean Louis Prévost and Jules Cotard in France (1865).

By the beginning of the 19th century, the clinical–anatomic method had spread from Italy to other countries but only at the end of the 19th century did authors begin to emphasize the relationship between arterial vascularization, brain lesions, and corresponding clinical features.

Jean-Martin Charcot (1825–1893) taught anatomic pathology before being nominated to the world's first chair of neurology. In 1862, Charcot and his friend Edmé Félix Alfred Vulpian (1826–1887) became directors of clinics at La Salpêtrière. The work of Charcot is widely recognized for its impact on neurology and psychology, but his contribution to vascular neurology remained small.

Between 1850 and 1900, the most common topics of study and interest were tabes and hysteria. A good example of the persisting relative disinterest in CVD by one of the most famous neurologists of this period is provided by Joseph Babinski (1857–1932). Only one paper focused on CVD, while the three others dealt with signs associated with hemiplegia. The critical trigger of the interest in CVD at this time was the description of specific brainstem syndromes. However, the underlying lesions were only rarely vascular, but were frequently tuberculomas, tumors, or abscesses. These reports stimulated prominent neurologists to study CVD cases from the angle of clinical–topographic correlations.

The turn of the 19th and 20th centuries saw the birth of the early generation of "vascular neurologists." Among them the Frenchman Charles Foix was particularly active. In the field of neurology, an interest in CVD as a distinct clinical entity took place at that time.

Foix is considered to be the first vascular neurologist for his work on the patterns of brain infarction in cerebral artery subdivision [10,11]. His work took a typical clinical–anatomic approach in an attempt to establish fine correlations between localization of parenchymal lesions and consequent clinical dysfunction.

The gradual evolution of knowledge during the 19th century was the result of work by isolated physicians or great names in pathology.

2.4. CVL Revolution in the 20th Century

After Charles Foix, interest in CVD gradually, though slowly, increased during the 20th century, especially in the 1940s and 1950s, with the advent of new diagnostic methods. Later work involved an increasing combination of morphological and physiopathological aspects followed by neuroimaging data.

In the 1960s, the Canadian Charles Miller Fisher (1913–2012) highlighted that a thromboembolic mechanism underlies the majority of ischemic CVLs and that the origin of thrombus derives from the heart or from a proximal arterial lesion [12]. He described the association of the lacunar lesion with specific neurological manifestations allowing the diagnosis of this type of CVD, very common in the decades before these ischemic lesions became visible on brain imaging studies.

The history of 20th century medicine relative to CVD/CVLs is fundamentally the result of the technical development in diagnostics [13].

3. Pathology of Cerebrovascular Lesions

CVLs result from the impaired function of the central nervous system vessels, divided into hemorrhagic, ischemic, or mixed. CVLs usually occur with sudden onset due to bursting of the cerebral arteries (hemorrhagic lesion) or/and occlusion by a thrombus or other particles (ischemic lesion); this results in focal brain dysfunction.

Critical advances in the study of CVLs came from pathologists such as Karl von Rokitansky (1804–1878) and Rudolf Ludwig Virchow.

In the 19th century, CVD became established as a scientific concept, and so medicine was included in the natural sciences. Working in Vienna, Karl von Rokitansky used post-mortem examination to document observations which aided future clinical diagnoses. The pathoanatomist Karl von Rokitansky, together with Joseph Škoda (1805–1881), developed the II. Viennese School, known as the "young Viennese School". The first volume of Rokitansky's "Compendium of General Pathological Anatomy" was published in Berlin in 1846, where a group of dedicated young physicians was particularly interested in "thinking cellularly" [14].

Arterial thrombosis and embolism were described by Rudolf Virchow who observed the interaction among blood and the arterial inner wall [9], and the results of interruption of blood flow to a parenchyma. He was also the first to use the term "ischemia".

He revived the term "arteriosclerosis" for the development of a thrombosis on the arterial wall, which had initially been employed by Jean Georges Chrétien Frédéric Martin Lobstein (1777–1835) in 1829, and furthermore demonstrated that portions of a thrombosis could detach from the wall and be carried in circulation as an "embolus" (also his term) [15].

Rudolf Virchow observed thrombosis secondary to arteriosclerosis, and local embolism caused by clots from the heart in patients with lower limb gangrene [16]. He extrapolated that a similar event in the brain could lead to cerebral softening. In 1856, he reported carotid thrombosis with ipsilateral blindness. Rudolf Virchow considered "arteriosclerosis" as "simple fat metamorphosis," and a frequent change in the blood vessel walls. Through Virchow's investigations, inflammation was universally considered as the principal etiological cause of arteriosclerosis, and this has been confirmed recently.

Virchow's studies were pursued by Julius Cohnheim (1839–1884), one of his students. When "cerebral vascular lesion" is used as an academic alternative for "stroke", the reference is to Cohnheim's theory derived from his experiments of arterial injection of wax globules embolizing in a frog's tongue. These observations suggested that arterial blockage and reduced blood flow to brain areas caused softenings, and that this confirmed Cohnheim's proposal that the lesions were infarctions [17]. Such embolization produced either no injury or two types of lesions, which for almost a century have been defined as "ischemic necrosis" and "hemorrhagic infarct" [17].

A great advance in the 1840s was due to Karl von Rokitansky who insisted on the association of hemorrhagic apoplexy with heart disease [18]. Various "apoplexies" were thought to be due to right ventricle congestion or dilatation. Hemorrhage may have been associated with left ventricle hypertrophy and, therefore, to an increased "impulse". Arterial hypertension had not been taken seriously at that time. What is more, fragile arterial walls were thought to provide to hemorrhagic lesion, either singly or together with these two aspects. Finally, it was believed that an "anomalous condition of the blood" existed, which corresponded to "arteriosclerosis". Von Rokitansky believed that artery "ossification" derived from "the accumulation of an inner membrane upon the vessel by deposition from arterial blood," and that the vessel wall absorbed a chemical substance in the blood, leading to fatty streaks [19].

4. Pathophysiology of Cerebrovascular Lesions

The pathophysiology of ischemic/hemorrhagic CVL results in oxygen-depleted focal cerebral nerve cells. The corresponding vascular territory is functionally disturbed and dies if circulation is not immediately reperfused. The pathogenesis of ischemic CVLs is multifactorial and the inflammatory process is a key component in CVL pathogenesis [20].

4.1. CVLs Pathophysiology from the 19th to 20th Centuries

The term apoplexy occurs in Hippocrates' aphorism "Unusual bouts of numbness and anesthesia are signs of impending apoplexy".

Apoplexy was described as a sudden and generalized brain disorder. Apoplexy pathogenesis was defined by means of the humoral theory—that is, the balance between the four humors, blood, phlegm, black and yellow bile. It was frequently thought to be caused by a cluster of black bile within the cerebral arterial vessels, thus blocking the passage of spirits animated from the ventricles, with anatomy playing almost no role [21]. In ancient times, medicine was closely linked to religion, without arousing much scientific interest.

During the Renaissance, Leonardo da Vinci (1452–1519), one of the best known and most famous anatomists, reported and illustrated the great neck vessels.

Indeed, Leonardo realized that neck compression (strangulation) led to rapid loss of consciousness and, if continued for more than some minutes, resulted in death from cerebral blood vessel compression [22].

From the end of the 19th century onwards, the scientific knowledge of medicine represents a branch of knowledge linked to the natural sciences. In this period, the possible correlation between cerebrovascular–anatomical lesions and some neurological manifestations or specific diseases are researched, and the diagnosis of electrophysiological and imaging techniques are improved.

In 1905, Hans Chiari (1851–1916), and some years later, Hunt, Moniz, and Hultquist, among others, recognized the possible correlation of carotid artery disease and CVD. Hans Chiari, working in Prague, observed thrombus superimposed upon ulcerated carotid artery atherosclerotic plaques in 7 out of 400 patients in consecutive autopsies [23]. There were four cases of cerebral embolism, and so Chiari hypothesized that embolic material could become detached from carotid artery plaques and determine brain damage such as CVD. Chiari was the first to correlate carotid occlusive disease with neurological symptoms.

In 1914, James Ramsay Hunt (1872–1937) described the clinical characteristics of 20 hemiplegia patients but without supplying autopsy data. Once again, he stressed the importance of extracranial artery blockage in CVD. Hunt realized that partial and complete innominate and carotid artery occlusions could be the vascular cause of cerebral syndromes; therefore, he used the expression "cerebral intermittent claudication". Furthermore, he emphasized "the occurrence of unilateral vascular changes, pallor or atrophy of the optic disk with contralateral hemiplegia" in carotid artery obstruction and proposed that "the cerebral lesions in most CVD victims could be the effect and not the cause" [24,25].

At the end of the 19th and early-20th centuries, the relationship between arterial encephalic vascularization and CVLs began to be understood [26]. Between the 1920s and 1970s, the pathophysiological knowledge of CVLs improved thanks to work by the Frenchman Charles Foix and the Canadian Charles Miller-Fisher [27].

In the same period, attention began to be focused on how the brain works, including its vascularization. Charles Foix is remembered for his CVD studies, with particular regard to posterior circulation disease. He paid particular attention to clinical–anatomical correlation, trying to find a relationship between CVL and clinical signs [28].

Foix's work dealt with an analysis of the anatomical regions and vascular structures of each branch, providing a description of the softening distribution and relative accompanying neurological manifestations.

In 1895, the revolutionary discovery of X-rays by Wilhelm Roentgen (1845–1923) contributed to a deepened knowledge of CVD and CVLs [29]. Wilhelm Roentgen assigned the name of his discovery X-rays, since the nature of these rays was unknown. Subsequently, one of his pupils, Max von Laue (1879–1960), demonstrated that they had the same electromagnetic nature as light, but differed only in the higher frequency of their vibration.

X-ray techniques continued to improve, and on 7th July 1927, the Portuguese Antonio Egas Moniz (1874–1955) described the first use of sodium iodide as a contrast medium in cerebral angiography at the Societé de Neurologie in Paris [30]. This breakthrough in CVD knowledge allows us to identify the affected vessel prior to surgical procedure [31].

Raymond Adams (1911–2008) and Charles Kubik (1891–1982) annotated the clinical findings and showed both the location of arterial occlusions and the resulting brain and cerebellar lesions [32]. They indicated morphological distinctions between thrombosis and embolism: "Thrombosis of the basilar artery could usually be recognized at a glance. The thrombosed portion of the vessel was distended, firm, and rigid and the thrombus could not be displaced by pressure. In embolism, the embolus was usually lodged in the distal portion of the basilar artery" [33].

Subsequently, Miller Fisher analyzed the artery pathology underlying lacunar lesions, cerebral hemorrhages, and carotid artery occlusions. In one of his works, Fisher highlighted the correlation between carotid artery occlusion in the neck and CVD diagnosis [34]. Further lacunar CVD studies and associated neurological diseases have allowed for the clinical diagnosis of these frequent and common ischemic CVLs decades before lesions were revealed by neuroimaging studies, thereby facilitating treatment [35,36].

Between the 19th and 20th centuries the pathophysiology of CVLs resulted from (i) experimental laboratory models; (ii) animal models of ischemic CVD; (iii) brain autopsies and anatomical preparations; (iv) electroencephalographic examinations; (v) X-ray techniques. Correlations between vascular and clinical anatomy became increasingly important. Animal models played a role in developing improved CVD prevention and treatment through the investigation of the pathophysiology of different CVD subtypes and by testing promising treatments before human trials began.

The pathophysiological basis of CVLs remained unclear until the 1960s, when Charles Miller Fisher carried out several autopsy studies on CVD patient brains. He described CVL pathological features in different nervous system areas such as thalamic and cerebellar hemorrhage lesion, lateral medullary infarction, and inflammatory CVLs. He found that the vessels exhibiting segmental arteriolar disorganization correlated with vessel enlargement, hemorrhage, and fibrinoid deposition.

This phenomenon has been termed "lipohyalinosis" to characterize the microvascular mechanism that generates small subcortical infarcts without a convincing embolic source. Notable progress has been made in understanding lipoyalinosis and lacunar stroke since Fisher's early studies.

Herein, we review the phenomenon of lipohyalinosis in relation to early concepts of cerebral small vessel disease [37]. Specific cerebral ischemia evolves through a phase of acute encephalomalacia, where alternating cellular swelling and shrinkage determines morphologic change. Leukocytic inflammation follows for three to four days after arterial occlusion and then after about the 10th day of resolution begins [38].

At the end of the 20th century, CVD animal models contributed to improved knowledge of different CVL pathophysiology, despite important differences between rodent and human cerebrovascular anatomy (brain dimensions, perforating artery length and structure, and gray to white matter ratio) [39].

4.2. Introducing Etiological Classification

By the beginning of the 19th century, the terms thrombosis, embolism, arteriosclerosis, and lacune to indicate CVL etiology were introduced, but atherosclerosis carotid disease was recognized later.

4.2.1. Thrombosis, Embolism Infarction and Arteriosclerosis

Thrombosis and embolism were first recognized by Rudolf Virchow to describe the relevant interaction between blood and arterial damage [9]. Virchow documented the consequences of blocking blood flow to a parenchymal or tissue and named this process "ischemia" (Schiller, 1970; Nuland, 1993; Reese, 1998).

At the beginning of the 19th century research began to concentrate on vascular alterations. In 1829, Jean Lobstein proposed the term "arteriosclerosis" in his unfinished four-volume treatise "Traité d'Anatomie Pathologique" [40].

In the middle of the 19th century, cellular inflammatory changes in atherosclerotic vessel walls were described by Rudolf Virchow and Karl von Rokitansky who represented two opposing schools of thought [41,42].

By 1848, Rudolf Virchow had shown that "thrombosis", his term, was due to masses in the blood vessels (Virchow, 1856; Pearce, 2002). He identified three principal predisposing factors for venous thrombosis, now known as Virchow's triad (irregularity of the vessel wall lumen, reduced blood flow, and hyper-coagulability).

Virchow reintroduced the definition "arteriosclerosis", initially used by Lobstein in 1829, to indicate that portions of a thrombosis could separate and form an "embolus" (also his term) [2]. Virchow noted thrombosis secondary to arteriosclerosis, and local embolism caused by clots from the heart in patients with lower limb gangrene. He considered "arteriosclerosis" as "simple fat metamorphosis," and that it was one of the most common changes in blood vessels.

Through Virchow's investigations, inflammation was widely recognized as the principal etiological cause of arteriosclerosis, which has been confirmed in recent decades.

4.2.2. Lacunar Infarction

Introduced initially in 1838 by Amédée Dechambre (1812–1886), the term "lacune" referred to a small cavity that remains after a small CVD [43]. This term is an uncommon example of an introduction of a French term which has remained unchanged in English. It derives from the Latin lacuna and it refers to an "empty space." In 1843, Charles Louis Maxime Durand-Fardel (1815–1899) described in more detail the finding of "lacunes" such as small healed brain attacks [44].

Durand-Fardel defined a lacune as a small cavity in the brain "without any change in consistency or color from which it was possible to remove a little cellular tissue containing very small vessels with a thin forceps". His objective was to distinguish "lacuna" from hemorrhage and large infarct. The issue as to whether lacunes were residual from a hemorrhage or an infarct led to a vehement argument between Rochoux and Durand-Fardel in 1844. Further advances on lacunes were not obtained during the next 50 years.

Pierre Marie, a devoted pupil of Jean-Marin Charcot, who became his third successor to the chair of Clinique des Maladies du Système Nerveux at La Salpêtrière, published his paper "Des foyer lacunaires de désintégration et les différents autres états cavitaires du cerveau" in 1901, in which he concluded that lacunes were small softenings caused by atherosclerosis, and were different from état criblé and "état vermoulu". He also declared that some lacunes which contained a patent blood vessel were due to a perivascular space dilation and ruined the contiguous brain parenchyma by "destructive vaginalitis".

When the term lacune was first described, its underlying pathophysiology was unclear. In the 1960s, Charles Miller-Fisher [35] performed autopsy studies that showed that vessels supplying lacunes displayed segmental arteriolar disorganization. He reintroduced Durand-Fardel's term for lacune as "small, deep cerebral infarct". Since then, there have been few attempts to render this pathological description consistent with modern mechanisms of cerebral small vessel disease [45].

4.2.3. Atherosclerotis Carotid Disease

Atherosclerosis has not recently developed in the last few centuries. It was present as degenerative modifications in the arterial walls of Egyptian mummies [46,47]. Ancient Egyptian atherosclerosis morphology does not differ from the phenomenon seen today in vascular surgery and pathoanatomic specimens.

Adolf Kussmaul (1822–1902) in 1872 and Franz Penzoldt (1849–1927) in 1881 reported thrombosis of carotid artery in the neck in patients with ipsilateral eye blindness and contralateral hemiplegia [48,49]. In 1875, William Richard Gowers (1845–1915) reported a patient with blindness and contralateral hemiplegia and mitral stenosis [50]. In the patient's autopsy findings, emboli were found in the central and retinal cerebral arteries, originating from clots in the auricular appendages. For more than a century, the cerebral embolic genesis was related to the heart and only since 1960 has it been considered the embolic source from the extracranial arterial.

Similarly, the term cerebral thrombosis remained well-entrenched as a synonym for cerebral infarction without cardiac embolism. It was generally assumed that arterial disease involved intracranial vessels, although in 1905 Hans Chiari [23] had emphasized the association of extracranial carotid disease with CVD.

In 1910, the German chemist Windaus demonstrated that atherosclerotic plaques were made up of calcified connective tissue and cholesterol [51]. Soon after, Nikolai Anitschkow and Semen Chaltow managed to induce atherosclerosis in rabbits by feeding them a cholesterol-rich diet, thus definitely identifying a classical risk factor for progression of atherosclerotic mechanisms [52].

The pathogenetic mechanism of atherosclerosis remained unclear and classical analyses did not attribute great importance to inflammatory–immunological processes as possible pathogenetic factors [53]. The inflammatory process has been identified as playing a fundamental part in atherogenesis.

5. Perspectives for the 21st Century

Multiple biological systems are involved in CVL pathogenesis, and future research should aim to pinpoint potential interactions among all these mechanisms in order to develop therapies for the prevention of CVD. The increase in CVL pathogenetic knowledge derives from (i) anatomopathological studies of fatal head injuries; (ii) neuroprotection laboratory and animal experiments; (iii) cerebral angiography studies; (iv) static or functional neuroimaging and related imaging techniques.

Current knowledge of CVL pathophysiological mechanisms is derived from the critical activity of the 19th century physicians who managed to confute all the deceptive and constricting beliefs that had existed for many centuries.

Funding: This research received no external funding.

Conflicts of Interest: The author declare no conflict of interest.

References

1. Safavi-Abbasi, S.; Reis, C.; Talley, M.C.; Theodore, N.; Nakaji, P.; Spetzler, R.F.; Preul, M.C. Rudolf Ludwig Karl Virchow: Pathologist, physician, anthropologist, and politician. Implications of his work for the understanding of cerebrovascular pathology and stroke. *Neurosurg. Focus* **2006**, *20*, E1. [PubMed]
2. Paciaroni, M.; Bogousslavsky, J. How did stroke become of interest to neurologists? A slow 19th century saga. *Neurology* **2009**, *73*, 724–728. [CrossRef] [PubMed]
3. Karenberg, A. Historic review: Select chapters of a history of stroke. *Neurol. Res. Pract.* **2020**, *2*, 34. [PubMed]
4. Garrison, F.H. *History of Neurology*; Revised and Enlarged by LC McHenry Jr.; Charles C Thomas: Springfield, IL, USA, 1969.
5. Platter, F. *Praxeos seu de Cognoscendis, Praedicendis, Praecavendis Curandisque Affectibus Homini Incommodantibus Tractatus Tres. Basel 1602–1608*; Translated into English under the title: A Golden Practice of Physick; Peter Cole: London, UK, 1662.
6. Ghosh, S.K. Giovanni Battista Morgagni (1682–1771): Father of pathologic anatomy and pioneer of modern medicine. *Anat. Sci. Int.* **2017**, *92*, 305–312. [PubMed]

7. Morgagni, G.B. *De Sedibus et Causis Morborum per Anatomen Indigatis Libri Quinque*; ex Typographica Remondiana: Venice, Italy, 1761.
8. Rochoux, J.A. *Recherches sur l'Apoplexie*; Chez Méquignon-Marvis: Paris, Franch, 1814.
9. Virchow, R.L.K. *Gesammelte Abhandlungen zur wissen-schaftlichen Medizin*; Meidinger Sohn & Co.: Frankfurt, Germany, 1856; pp. 219–732.
10. Foix, C.; Chavany, H.; Hillemand, P.; Schiff-Wertheimer, M. Oblitération de l'artére choroïdienne antérieure: Ramollissement de son territoire cérébral: Hémiplégie, hémianesthésie et hémianopsie. *Bull. Soc. Ophtalmol. Fr.* **1925**, *27*, 221–223.
11. Foix, C.; Masson, A. Le syndrome de l'artére cérébrale posteérieure. *Presse Meéd* **1923**, *31*, 361–365.
12. Paciaroni, M.; Bogousslavsky, J. The history of stroke and cerebrovascular disease. *Handb. Clin. Neurol.* **2008**, *92*, 3–28.
13. Marshall, J.; Shaw, D.A. The natural history of cerebrovascular disease. *Br. Med. J.* **1959**, *1*, 1614–1617. [CrossRef]
14. Becker, V. Rokitansky and Virchow: Throes about the scientific term of disease. *Wien. Med. Wochenschr.* **2005**, *155*, 463–467. [CrossRef]
15. Lobstein, J.F.M. *Traité d'Anatomie Pathologique*; Levrault: Paris, Franch, 1829.
16. Virchow, R.L.K. Ueber die acute Entzűndung der Arterien. *Arch. Pathol. Anat.* **1847**, *1*, 272–378.
17. Cohnheim, J. *Untersuchungen Ueber die Embolischen Prozesse*; Hirschwald: Berlin, Germany, 1872.
18. von Rokitansky, C. *A Manual of Pathological Anatomy (1824–1844), Vol. III*; Sydenham Society: London, UK, 1856; pp. 399–419.
19. Whisnant, J.P. Cerebrovascular Diseases: Natural History. *Public Health Monogr.* **1966**, *76*, 9–21.
20. Duyckaerts, C.; Hauw, J.J. Pathology and pathophysiology of brain ischaemia. *Neuroradiology* **1985**, *27*, 460–467.
21. Clarke, E. Apoplexy in the Hippocratic writings. *Bull. Hist. Med.* **1963**, *37*, 301–314.
22. McCurdy, E. *Leonardo da Vinci: The Notebooks: Arranged, Rendered and Introduced by McCurdy*; G. Braziller: New York, NY, USA, 1955.
23. Chiari, H. Ueber Verhalten des Teilungswinkels der Carotis communis bei der Endarteritis chronica deformans. *Verh. Dtsch. Ges. Pathol.* **1905**, *9*, 326.
24. Thompson, J.E. The evolution of surgery for the treatment and prevention of stroke. *Stroke* **1996**, *27*, 1427–1434.
25. Hunt, J.R. The role of the carotid arteries in the causation of vascular lesions of the brain, with remarks on certain special features of the symptomatology. *Am. J. Med. Sci.* **1914**, *147*, 704–713. [CrossRef]
26. Warlow, C.P.; Dennis, M.S.; van Gijn, J. Development of knowledge concerning cerebrovascular disease. In *Stroke: A Practical Guide to Management*; Blackwell Science: Oxford, UK, 2001.
27. Fields, W.S.; Lemak, N.A. *A History of Stroke. Its Recognition and Treatment*; Oxford University Press: New York, NY, USA, 1989.
28. Hillemand, P. Charles Foix et son oeuvre 1882–1927. *Clin. Med.* **1976**, *11*, 269–287.
29. Roentgen, W.K. On a new kind of rays. *Science* **1896**, *3*, 227–231. [CrossRef]

30. Moniz, E. L'encéphalographie arterielle, son importance dans la localisation des tumeurs cé ré brales. *Rev. Neurol.* **1927**, *2*, 72–90.
31. Estol, C.J. Dr C. Miller Fisher and the history of carotid artery disease. *Stroke* **1996**, *27*, 559–566.
32. Caplan, L.R. Posterior circulation ischemia: Then, now, and tomorrow. The Thomas Willis Lecture 2000. *Stroke* **2000**, *31*, 2011–2023. [PubMed]
33. Kubic, C.S.; Adams, R.D. Occlusion of the basilar artery: A clinical and pathological study. *Brain* **1946**, *69*, 73–121. [CrossRef]
34. Fisher, C.M. Occlusion of the internal carotid artery. *Arch. Neurol.* **1951**, *65*, 346–377. [CrossRef] [PubMed]
35. Fisher, C.M. Lacunes: Small, deep cerebral infarcts. *Neurology* **1965**, *15*, 774–784. [PubMed]
36. Fisher, C.M. Capsular infarcts: The underlying vascular lesions. *Arch. Neurol.* **1979**, *36*, 65–73.
37. Regenhardt, R.W.; Das, A.S.; Lo, E.H.; Caplan, L.R. Advances in Understanding the Pathophysiology of Lacunar Stroke: A Review. *JAMA Neurol.* **2018**, *75*, 1273–1281.
38. Garcia, J.H. The neuropathology of stroke. *Hum. Pathol.* **1975**, *6*, 583–598.
39. Krafft, P.R.; Bailey, E.L.; Lekic, T.; Rolland, W.B.; Altay, O.; Tang, J.; Wardlaw, J.M.; Zhang, J.H.; Sudlow, C.L.M. Etiology of Stroke and Choice of Models. *Int. J. Stroke* **2012**, *7*, 398–406.
40. Millonig, G.; Schwentner, C.; Mueller, P.; Mayerl, C.; Wick, G. The vascular-associated lymphoid tissue: A new site of local immunity. *Curr. Opin. Infect. Dis.* **2001**, *12*, 547–553.
41. Rokitansky, C. *A Manual of Pathological Anatomy*; Blanchard and Lea: Philadelphia, PA, USA, 1855.
42. Virchow, R. *Cellular Pathology as Based Upon Physiological and Pathological Histology (English Translation of Second German Edition)*; JB, Lippincott: Philadelphia, PA, USA, 1971.
43. Dechambre, A. Mémoire sur lacurabilité du ramollissement cérébral. *Gaz. Médicale De Paris* **1938**, *6*, 305–314.
44. Durand-Fardel, C.L.M. *Traité du Ramollissement du Cerveau*; J.B. Bailliére: Paris, Franch, 1843.
45. Regenhardt, R.W.; Das, A.S.; Ohtomo, R.; Lo, E.H.; Ayata, C.; Gurol, M.E. Pathophysiology of Lacunar Stroke: History's Mysteries and Modern Interpretations. *J. Stroke Cerebrovasc. Dis.* **2019**, *28*, 2079–2097.
46. Ruffer, M.A. On arterial lesions found in Egyptian mummies (1580B.C.—525A.D.). *J. Pathol. Bacteriol.* **1911**, *15*, 453–462. [CrossRef]
47. Sandison, A.T. Degenerative vascular disease in the Egyptian mummy. *Med. Hist.* **1962**, *6*, 77–81. [CrossRef]
48. Kussmaul, A. Zwei Falle von spontaner allmaliger Verschliessung grosser Halsarterienstamme. *Dtsch Klein* **1872**, *24*, 461–465.
49. Penzoldt, F. Ueber Thrombose (autochtone oder embolische) der Carotis. *Dtsch. Arch. Klein Med.* **1881**, *28*, 80–93.
50. Gowers, W.R. On a case of simultaneous embolism of central retinal and middle cerebral arteries. *Lancet* **1875**, *2*, 794–796. [CrossRef]

51. Anitschkow, N.; Chalatow, S. Ueber experimentelle Cholesterinsteatose und ihre Bedeutung für die Entstehung einiger pathologischer Prozesse. *Zentralbl. Allg. Pathol.* **1913**, *24*, 1–9.
52. Windaus, A. Ueber den Gehalt normaler und atheromatoeser Aorten an Cholesterol and Cholesterinester. *Zeitschrift. Physiol. Chem.* **1910**, *67*, 174–176. [CrossRef]
53. Mayerl, C.; Lukasser, M.; Sedivy, R.; Niederegger, H.; Seiler, R.; Wick, G. Atherosclerosis research from past to present on the track of two pathologists with opposing views, Carl von Rokitansky and Rudolf Virchow. *Virchows Arch.* **2006**, *449*, 96–103.

© 2023 by the author. Licensee MDPI, Basel, Switzerland. This article is an open access article distributed under the terms and conditions of the Creative Commons Attribution (CC BY) license (http://creativecommons.org/licenses/by/4.0/).

History of Cardiac Embolism

Giacomo Staffolani, Michela Giustozzi and Maurizio Paciaroni

Abstract: From 1742, the first time Gerhard van Swieten postulated that embolism might arise inside the heart chambers and great vessels, another century was needed before that clinicians became accustomed to the concept that an embolism can lead to an occlusion of a brain artery. In fact, in 1875, Gowers described a case of blindness and contralateral hemiplegia in a patient with mitral stenosis. At autopsy, emboli were found in the middle cerebral artery and in the central retinal artery. Specifically, the emboli were found to originate from clots on the auricular appendices. Subsequently, in 1954, Fisher demonstrated that a thromboembolic mechanism underlies most ischemic strokes and that the source of thrombus might be the heart rather than a proximal arterial lesion. He suggested that the embolus might have arisen after myocardial infarction, in the fibrillating atrial appendage. In 1977, a necropsy study provided additional evidence supporting the role of atrial fibrillation as a crucial cause of cerebral embolism which was later confirmed by large epidemiological studies. Finally, in the first part of the 1990's, several studies reported that oral anticoagulants consistently reduced the risk of stroke in patients with atrial fibrillation. Oral anticoagulants currently remain the most powerful stroke prevention strategy available for patients with atrial fibrillation.

1. History of Embolism

Gerhard van Swieten (1742) was a precursor in postulating embolism arising inside the heart chambers and great vessels: *"It has been established by many observations that these polyps occasionally attach themselves as excrescences to the columnae carneae of the heart, and perhaps separate from it and are propelled, along with the blood, into the pulmonary artery or the aorta, and its branches ... were they thrown into the carotid or vertebral arteries, could disturb—or if they completely blocked all approach of arterial blood to the brain—utterly abolish all functions of the brain".* [1]

Virchow (1847), a century later, observed embolism (a term newly introduced in the medical language by him) in patients with gangrene of the lower extremities as the cause of clots formed in the heart [2]. He proposed that the same phenomenon could be the cause of cerebral softening: *"In contrast to that kind of obliterating clot we find another kind. Here there is either no essential change in the vessel wall and its surroundings, or this is ostensibly secondary. I feel perfectly justified in claiming that these clots never originated in the local circulation but that they are torn off at a distance and carried along in the blood stream as far as they can go".* [3]

Sometime later, William Senhouse Kirkes published one of the first descriptions of infective endocarditis associated with cerebral embolism, thus providing its first extensive clinical and pathological illustration [4].

Within a short period of time, clinicians became accustomed to the concept of embolic occlusion.

Virchow's efforts in the vascular area were continued and crowned by his exceptional student Julius Cohnheim, whose theory of ischemic necrosis and hemorrhagic infarction was based on the experimental evidence of injecting wax emboli into test animal's tongue and observing the damage to the vascular endothelium. In the same years, Carl Rokitansky introduced a novel concept: the close mechanical association between hemorrhagic apoplexy and heart disease. In his four-volume manual published in 1856, he stated that many apoplexies were determined by congestion or dilatation of the right ventricle [3].

In 1875, W.R. Gowers presented a case of blindness and contralateral hemiplegia in a patient affected by mitral stenosis. Postmortem examination revealed the presence of emboli in the middle cerebral artery and in the central retinal artery; it was speculated that the clots arose from the auricular appendage associated with mitral stenosis [5]. In Osler's time (late 19th and early 20th centuries), it became well accepted that brain embolism had its source in diseases of the heart, with particular reference to bacterial endocarditis and rheumatic heart disease with mitral stenosis [6].

2. The Role of Atrial Fibrillation

Atrial fibrillation has been known for decades, but was established as a clinical entity in 1909 by Sir Thomas Lewis, who captured it on an ECG and studied the mechanism of conduction, noting that atrial fibrillation was "contiously and extremely irregular". He called it a "common clinical condition", establishing it as a clinical entity [7].

Around the midpoint of the 20th century, cardiologists started to suggest that atrial fibrillation was an important precursor of cerebral embolism in patients with rheumatic mitral stenosis [8]. Atrial stasis as a result of mitral stenosis, and often in the presence of AF, has long been recognized as a predisposing factor to thrombus formation; investigators begin to question if AF played a role in the occurrence of systemic embolism including stroke [6].

In 1949, Miller Fisher was among the first academics to imply a role for atrial fibrillation in causing brain embolism, even in the absence of endocarditis or rheumatic heart disease [6]: in his memoirs, Fisher stated *"I had the opportunity to examine the cerebral arteries before slicing 3 brains that had large hemorrhagic infarcts. The basal vessels were empty of thrombus. People were signing out these cases as cerebral artery thrombosis – but pathologically there was no thrombus. Afterwards, I looked up the records on these 3 cases and they had all been in atrial fibrillation and the general autopsy had shown infarcts in the spleen and kidneys. I speculated that they might be cases of embolism from the heart."* [9].

However, the current thinking among cardiologists did not change for more than twenty years: emboli infrequently arose from a fibrillating heart without rheumatic disease, and so AF, in absence of RHD, was considered a benign condition [6,10].

In spite of the common knowledge of that time, the evidence based on pathological, clinical and epidemiological studies kept on accumulating: in 1970, Coulshed et al. recognized the presence of atrial fibrillation as the critical factor that leads to systemic embolism in patients with mitral valve disease. Among the population affected by mitral stenosis, the incidence of systemic embolism (embolic stroke included) was three times higher in those with atrial fibrillation than in those with synus rhythm [11]. Szekely reported that systemic embolism occurred more than seven times as frequently in patients with mitral valve disease who had atrial fibrillation [12].

In 1977, a necropsy study provided additional evidence supporting the role of lone atrial fibrillation as an important cause of embolism. The study took into account 333 autopsy patients with atrial fibrillation associated with different kinds of heart disease: the results displayed a high incidence rate of embolism in patients with AF, irrespective of the presence or absence of mitral valve disease [10].

The very next year, data from the prospective epidemiological Framingham Heart Study became available: Wolf and colleagues compared the incidence of stroke in people with and without chronic atrial fibrillation. In total, 345 documented strokes had occurred after 24 years of follow-up: 27 in subjects with chronic AF, 7 with RHD, and 20 with non-rheumatic AF.

In persons with AF associated with rheumatic heart disease, there was a 17.6-fold increase in the incidence of stroke, and in those with AF in the absence of valvular disease, there was a 5.6-fold increase in stroke incidence, even when age and hypertensive status were taken into account [13].

After a follow-up of 34 years, 572 stroke events had occurred and the presence of atrial fibrillation was associated with a near five-fold increase in the 2-year age-adjusted incidence of stroke compared with its absence. Since cardiac conditions often coexist, even at a subclinical level, the increased risk of stroke associated with atrial fibrillation was also demonstrated in the presence of overt coronary heart disease (more than two-fold excess in men, near five-fold excess in women) and cardiac failure (two-fold excess).

While AF-related risk of stroke increased significantly with age, the attributable risk of stroke derived from other cardiovascular diseases was not affected by age [14].

Those epidemiological data were also supported by a comprehensive study in which 154 patients with anterior-circulation stroke and atrial fibrillation were evaluated for alternative determinants of stroke by carotid angiography or noninvasive carotid imaging; lacunar infarction was excluded by computed tomography. Atrial fibrillation emerged as the sole stroke mechanism in 76% of these cases [15].

3. Anticoagulation

McLean discovered the anticoagulant effect of heparin in 1915 while he was trying to extract a procoagulant from dog liver. It was successfully isolated in the early 1930s and was first administered to people in 1935. By the early 1940s, heparin was effectively used in patients and its efficacy in thromboembolic pathologies was confirmed by clinical trials.

In 1993, while studying a hemorrhagic disease affecting cattle, Link identified dicumarol from spoiled sweet clover hay as the agent responsible for sweet clover disease, a hemorrhagic disorder in cattle [16].

In late 1940 dicumarol was given to human volunteers, and in 1941, Dr. Wright became the first to use dicumarol therapeutically, immediately treating his thrombosis patients with success [17].

In 1994, a metanalysis of five RCTs by atrial fibrillation investigators showed that warfarin consistently reduced the risk of stroke by 68% in patients with atrial fibrillation, without virtually no increase in the frequency of major bleeding; people with lone atrial fibrillation had a low risk of stroke, which increased with advancing age [18].

These studies have established the role of anticoagulant therapy, which represents the single most powerful stroke prevention measure available. Taking into consideration the aging of the population and the improved survival of patients with heart diseases that predispose to atrial fibrillation (such as congestive heart failure and coronary heart disease), anticoagulation therapy continues to increase in importance in preventing cardioembolic stroke [19].

Author Contributions: The Authors have drafted the work or substantially revised it and have approved the submitted version. All authors have read and agreed to the published version of the manuscript.

Funding: this review received no external funding.

Conflicts of Interest: The Authors declare no conflict of interest.

References

1. van Swieten, G. *Of the Apoplexy, Palsy and Epilepsy. Commentaries on the Aphorisms of Dr Herman Boerhaave. Translation from Six Volumes (Lugduni Batavorum, J & H Verbeek, 1742–76)*; John & Paul Knapton: London, UK, 1754; Volume 10.
2. Paciaroni, M.; Bogousslavsky, J. Chapter 1 The history of stroke and cerebrovascular disease. In *Handbook of Clinical Neurology*; Elsevier: Amsterdam, The Netherlands, 2008; Volume 92, pp. 3–28.
3. Schiller, F. Concepts of stroke before and after Virchow. *Med. Hist.* **1970**, *14*, 115–131. [CrossRef] [PubMed]
4. Kirkes, W.S. Detachment of fibrinous deposits from the interior of the heart, and their mixture with the circulating blood. *Med. Chir. Trans. Lond.* **1852**, *35*, 281–324. [CrossRef] [PubMed]

5. Gowers, W.R. On a case of simultaneous embolism of central retinal and middle cerebral arteries. *Lancet* **1875**, *2*, 794–796. [CrossRef]
6. Caplan, L.R. Atrial Fibrillation, Past and Future: From a Stroke Non-Entity to an Over-Targeted Cause. *Cerebrovasc. Dis.* **2018**, *45*, 149–153. [CrossRef] [PubMed]
7. Fye, W.B. Tracing atrial fibrillation—100 years. *N. Engl. J. Med.* **2006**, *355*, 1412–1414. [CrossRef] [PubMed]
8. Harris, A.W.; Levine, S.A. Cerebral embolism in mitral stenosis. *Ann. Intern. Med.* **1941**, *15*, 637–643.
9. Fisher, C.M. *Memoirs of a Neurologist, vol 1*; Rutland Vermont, Sharp & Co. Printers: Rutland, VT, USA, 2006.
10. Hinton, R.C.; Kistler, J.P.; Fallon, J.T.; Friedlich, A.L.; Fisher, C.M. Influence of etiology of atrial fibrillation on incidence of systemic embolism. *Am. J. Cardiol.* **1977**, *40*, 509–513. [CrossRef] [PubMed]
11. Dalen, J.E. Atrial Fibrillation and Embolic Stroke. *Arch. Intern. Med.* **1991**, *151*, 1922–1924. [CrossRef] [PubMed]
12. Szekely, P. Systemic embolism and anticoagulant prophylaxis in rheumatic heart disease. *BMJ* **1964**, *1*, 209. [CrossRef] [PubMed]
13. Wolf, P.A.; Dawber, T.R.; Thomas, H.E., Jr.; Kannel, W.B. Epidemiologic assessment of chronic atrial fibrillation and risk of stroke: The Framingham study. *Neurology* **1978**, *28*, 973–977. [CrossRef] [PubMed]
14. Wolf, P.A.; Abbott, R.D.; Kannel, W.B. Atrial fibrillation as an independent risk factor for stroke: The Framingham Study. *Stroke* **1991**, *22*, 983–988. [CrossRef] [PubMed]
15. Bogousslavsky, J.; Van Melle, G.; Regli, F.; Kappenberger, L. Pathogenesis of anterior circulation stroke in patients with nonvalvular atrial fibrillation: The Lausanne Stroke Registry. *Neurology* **1990**, *40*, 1046–1050. [CrossRef] [PubMed]
16. Gómez-Outes, A.; Suárez-Gea, M.L.; Calvo-Rojas, G.; Lecumberri, R.; Rocha, E.; Pozo-Hernández, C.; Terleira-Fernández, A.I.; Vargas-Castrillón, E. Discovery of anticoagulant drugs: A historical perspective. *Curr. Drug. Discov. Technol.* **2012**, *9*, 83–104. [CrossRef] [PubMed]
17. Wright, I.S. Experiences with dicumarol in the treatment of coronary thrombosis. *Proc. Am. Fed. Clin. Res.* **1945**, *2*, 101. [PubMed]
18. Risk factors for stroke and efficacy of antithrombotic therapy in atrial fibrillation. Analysis of pooled data from five randomized controlled trials. *Arch. Intern. Med.* **1994**, *154*, 1449–1457.
19. Wolf, P.A. Awareness of the role of atrial fibrillation as a cause of ischemic stroke. *Stroke* **2014**, *45*, e19–e21. [CrossRef] [PubMed]

© 2023 by the authors. Licensee MDPI, Basel, Switzerland. This article is an open access article distributed under the terms and conditions of the Creative Commons Attribution (CC BY) license (http://creativecommons.org/licenses/by/4.0/).

History of "Lacunar Infarction"

Giacomo Baso and Leonardo Pantoni

Abstract: The concept of lacunar infarction has evolved over the last 200 years, from the first neuropathological observations to the current definition based on neuroimaging. In this chapter, the historical evolution of the definition of lacunar infarcts is reviewed, from the first original description by Amédée Dechambre to the detailed studies by Maxime Durand-Fardel and Virchow. The evolution of the pathogenetic and the etiological considerations from those of Binswanger, Alzheimer, and Pierre Marie to the memorable work of C. Miller Fisher is also revised. The critics of the lacunar hypothesis and the modern neuroimaging aspects are also considered.

1. Introduction

The modern concept of lacunar infarction is the result of a long succession of studies over the last 200 years [1]. Nowadays, lacunar infarctions are known to be small cystic cavities in the brain parenchyma caused by an ischemic insult in a territory perfused by a penetrating arteriole originating superficially from the superficial circulation as terminal vessels of medium-sized arteries, or deeper, from the large vessels of the Willis circle, the so-called "arterial perforators". By definition, lacunar infarctions have to be smaller than 15 mm and they represent small holes of encephalomalacia (i.e., lacunes). It is nowadays well known that lacunes can also result from small deep hemorrhages or correlate with isolated dilatation of the perivascular space [2].

2. The Historical Evolution of Lacunar Infarcts

2.1. Early Concepts

The first mention of lacunar infarction follows in time the early general descriptions, in 1820, of cerebral infarctions, named at that time "ramollissement du cerveau" or "cerebral softening" [3,4]. Eighteen years later, Amédée Dechambre provided the original description of lacunes, linking them to his name for years. As an intern at the Salpétriere Hospital in Paris, he was the first to study stroke survivors. He performed a brain autopsy, discovering many small lacunes of variable size and form. He identified them as the result of liquefaction and resorption of the infarct (cerebral softening). Maxime Durand-Fardel, the author of one of the first books on ischemic stroke ever published, independently postulated in 1843 the same origin of lacunes of Dechambre, distinguishing them from another type of parenchyma cavitation, the dilatation of the perivascular spaces, referred to as état criblé. Similar conclusions were achieved in the same years by the German pathologist Virchow [5]. In 1866, Laborde hypothesized that a lacune could be also the result of a small brain hemorrhage reabsorption. In 1894, Binswanger and Alzheimer described brains in which multiple lacunar infarctions were present more or less associated with cognitive decline. At the beginning of the 20th century, Compte observed multiple lacunes in patients with pseudobulbar palsy, and Thurel, in 1929, supposed lacunes as the most frequent etiology of this clinical picture. Independent of the works above described, in 1900, Pierre Marie provided a well-detailed clinical description, under the name of état lacunaire, of a set of recurrent motor deficit episodes, often with a partial resolution, followed by the onset of a clinical picture characterized by small-step gait, urinary incontinence, and pseudobulbar palsy. He also depicted some degree of global intellectual deterioration in these patients. Pierre Marie may be considered the first to have established the lacunar concept by associating the pathological and the clinical pictures. Together with Ferrand, he described a brain pathologic condition characterized by multiple lacunes, very similar to the arteriosclerotic brain atrophy depicted by Alzheimer and Binswanger. Despite what is reported above, in the following years, some confusion arose in the scientific community surrounding the concept of lacunes and their underlying etiology. Depré and Devaux's reported histological observations of lacunes, misinterpreting them as état criblé and therefore assigning them a non-ischemic origin [4]. In his publication in 1842, Durand called état criblé the perivascular spaces dilatation observed around cerebral arterioles in elderly patients, located in the context of white matter, and considered this picture as the result of vascular congestion. In 1920 C. and O. Vogt, even though they were the first to emphasize the "softening hypothesis", called status desintegrationis, as the union of the lacunar lesions in the globus pallidus and the striatum with dilatation of perivascular spaces. The confusion regarding lacunes was so pronounced that, in 1929, Thurel stated that the term état lacunaire should be used for the grey nuclei and that of état criblé for the centrum ovale and myelinated areas.

2.2. Lacunar Infarction in the 20th Century

The issue was solved only many years later by the seminal work of C. Miller Fisher. In 1965, he finally cleared the ambiguity by publishing a memorable paper [6], reporting on an outstanding series of 1042 consecutive brain examinations. A macroscopic search for lacunes, defined as irregular cavities between 0.5 and 15 mm in diameter, was performed through horizontal sections, registering location, size, and appearance. He described a characteristic pathology of vessels supplying the lacunar infarct's territory. The examination of these tiny arteries showed no occlusion at their origin. They had instead focal enlargements of the wall and small transmural hemorrhagic extravasations. He found that the vessel's lumen could also be obliterated by subintimal foam cells and that the walls of these vessels were filled with pink-staining fibrinoid material. Moreover, arteries could be replaced by connective tissue deposition, obliterating the usual vascular layers. He defined, respectively, these processes as segmental arterial disorganization, fibrinoid degeneration, and lipohyalinosis. These changes along the walls of the brain's small vessels, different from usual atheroma, led to the occlusion of a single penetrating artery, and then to an infarct in the referral vascular territory [7]. Thus, lacunes became the correlate of small deep cerebral infarcts, returning to Durand-Fardel's definition. He also described five classical lacunar syndromes, pure motor, ataxic hemiparesis, dysarthria-clumsy hand, pure sensory, and mixed sensorimotor [8].

All but three of the 114 patients with lacunes included in Fisher's review had hypertension [6]. In many of these patients, brain infarction developed during a period of high blood pressure levels, in an era in which clearly effective antihypertensive medications were not available. Additionally, Prineas and Marshall [9], followed by Cole and Yates [10], confirmed the role of hypertension, respectively in 1966 and 1967. Some years later, in 1982, J.P. Mohr deepened Fisher's pathological concepts [11]. In his work, fibrinoid necrosis affected arterioles and capillaries in a setting of extremely high blood pressure levels. Arterial wall thickness was increased, leading to damage to the autoregulation system of cerebrovascular afferents. According to his hypothesis, high pressure levels increase capillaries' hydrostatic pressure, damaging them irreversibly. Lipohyalinosis, instead, occurs after long exposure to non-malignant high blood pressure. In chronic hypertension, there are also tiny foci of atheromatous deposits, involving the walls of the penetrating arteries [11]. In consideration of that, Fisher and other researchers later postulated also a truly atherosclerotic pathway at the origin of lacunar infarction. It consists of little atherosclerotic plaques inside the small perforators, naming them microatheroma [12]. Hence, the lacunar hypothesis was founded, consisting of two parts. Firstly, symptomatic lacunes present with a limited number of distinct clinical lacunar syndromes. Secondly, lacunes are due to a specific disease of the penetrating arteries. If both conditions are respected, then the stroke has to be classified as caused by a "lacunar infarction" [13].

2.3. Lacunar Infarction beyond the Original Concept

In 1990, Millikan and Futrell [14] formally argued Fisher's lacunar hypothesis. In experimental models, rats with internal carotid photochemically induced damage showed microemboli dissemination to the brain, producing cavitary lesions similar to human lacunes. According to these authors, a lacunar syndrome should instead be considered the clinical result of a small subcortical infarct, and not a particular entity resulting from the combination of hypertension and small vessel disease. A few years later, to ensure the ability of a lacunar syndrome in predicting the radiologic presence of a lacunar infarction on brain imaging, the Northern Manhattan Stroke Study was settled [15]. In this study, a lacunar syndrome had a positive predictive value of 87% in detecting radiologic lacune, and a positive predictive value of 75% in predicting a final diagnosis of lacunar infarction. Notably, 25% of lacunar syndromes that were confirmed radiologically had a non-lacunar (i.e., not caused by small vessel disease) possible mechanism of infarction.

Futrell then developed the microembolic hypothesis. Together with the original observations based on rodent models, it was supposed that small infarcts could be the consequence of embolic occlusion originating from large arteries or from the heart [16]. Evidence supporting this theory was derived from primate models studies [17], but also from observational considerations that emerged from the analysis of data from trials on symptomatic internal carotid stenosis endarterectomies, in which some patients with ischemic lacunar infarction had a reduced stroke risk after vascular surgery of the symptomatic carotid [18].

These observations, therefore, expand the possible etiological mechanisms of lacunar infarction and are coupled with Fisher and Caplan's description of lacunar infarcts associated with atherosclerosis [19,20]. Atherosclerotic plaque lesions of major vessels could occlude the penetrating artery branches' orifices, a condition called intracranial branch atheromatous disease. Thus, also an atheroma originating in the parent artery could occlude the penetrating branches, a condition referred to as junctional atheromatous plaques [21].

3. The Current Role of Neuroimaging

The historical evolution of the concept of lacunar infarction has profoundly changed after the introduction of computed tomography (CT) and magnetic resonance imaging (MRI) in recent decades of the 20th century [22]. However, while neuroimaging has made small lesions of the brain visible in vivo, it has also introduced some problems such as the distinction between lacunar infarcts, lacunes due to old hemorrhages, and enlarged perivascular spaces. Historically, the first studies on CT scan detection were conducted in the 1980s [23,24]. When visible, lesions appear as punctuate areas of low density, whereas they transform into hypodense foci, of the same density of the cerebrospinal fluid. Detection rates were variable accordingly to clinical presentation, with global low sensitivity to acute small deep infarcts, especially in the first hours or when located in the posterior fossa [25]. Moreover, the smallest lesions of the posterior fossa were often not considered by researchers because only strokes revealed by classical lacunar syndrome were included, so a higher detection rate of pure motor stroke could be overestimated [26,27]. Indeed, a CT scan does not provide information about the age of lesions detected, unless serially repeated exams are used with evidence of a new lesion not visible in the previous scan [24]. MRI has strongly changed diagnostic capability since its introduction [28]. Even before diffusion imaging's advent, MRI showed higher sensitivity [29]. Among MRI sequences T2 (transverse relaxation time)-weighted appear superior to T1(longitudinal relaxation time)-weighted one [30]. Diffusion weighted imaging (DWI) finally showed the best performance, with hyperintense lesions together with restricted diffusion on apparent diffusion coefficient maps [31]. Notably, MRI acute appearance is strictly dependent on the sequence adopted. A slight hypointensity in T1, and hyperintensity in T2/Fluid-attenuated inversion recovery(FLAIR), with restricted diffusion in DWI and enhancement in fat suppressed T1-weighted gradient-echo sequence (T1C+) if acute or early subacute. Chronic lesions are isointense to cerebrospinal fluid independently from sequences. There is often a peripheral rim of marginal gliosis, hyperintense in T2/FLAIR sequences.

MRI is also able to distinguish between cavitated lesions due to ischemia, hemorrhage, or enlargement of perivascular spaces. The current history of lacunar infarcts has been characterized by the consensus paper published almost 10 years ago and aimed at defining neuroimaging standards for small vessel disease [32].

4. Conclusions

As outlined in this chapter, the definition of lacunar infarctions has evolved for a long time, and it is currently used both for lesions in the acute phase and for those in the chronic stage, according to technical information on the best neuroimaging acquisition techniques available.

Author Contributions: G.B., major role in drafting and editing the chapter; L.P. major role in drafting and editing the chapter. All authors have read and agreed to the published version of the manuscript.

Funding: This research received no external funding.

Conflicts of Interest: The authors declare no conflict of interest.

References

1. Paciaroni, M.; Bogousslavsky, J. Chapter 1—The history of stroke and cerebrovascular disease. In *Handbook of Clinical Neurology*; Fisher, M., Ed.; Elsevier: Amsterdam, The Netherlands, 2008; Volume 92, pp. 3–28, ISBN 9780444520036.
2. Derouesné, C.; Poirier, J. Les lacunes cerebrales: Un debat toujours d'actualite. *Rev. Neurol.* **1999**, *155*, 823–831.
3. Besson, G.; Hommel, M.; Perret, J. Historical aspects of the lacunar concept. *Cerebrovasc. Dis.* **1991**, *1*, 306–310. [CrossRef]
4. Román, G.C. On the history of lacunes, etat criblé, and the white matter lesions of vascular dementia. *Cerebrovasc. Dis.* **2002**, *13* (Suppl. 2), 1–6. [CrossRef] [PubMed]
5. Caplan, L.R. Penetrating arteries. In *Vertebrobasilar Ischemia and Hemorrhage*; Caplan, L.R., Ed.; Cambridge University Press: Cambridge, UK, 2015; pp. 369–420.
6. Fisher, C.M. Lacunes: Small, Deep Cerebral Infarcts. *Neurology* **1965**, *15*, 774–784. [CrossRef]
7. Fisher, C.M. The arterial lesions underlying lacunes. *Acta Neuropathol.* **1968**, *12*, 1–15. [CrossRef] [PubMed]
8. Fisher, C.M. Lacunar strokes and infarcts: A review. *Neurology* **1982**, *32*, 871–876. [CrossRef] [PubMed]
9. Prineas, J.; Marshall, J. Hypertension and cerebral infarction. *Br. Med. J.* **1966**, *1*, 14–17. [CrossRef] [PubMed]
10. Cole, F.M.; Yates, P. Intracerebral microaneurysms and small cerebrovascular lesions. *Brain* **1967**, *90*, 759–768. [CrossRef]

11. Mohr, J.P. Lacunes. *Stroke* **1982**, *13*, 3–11. [CrossRef]
12. De Jong, G.; Kessels, F.; Lodder, J. Two types of lacunar infarcts: Further arguments from a study on prognosis. *Stroke* **2002**, *33*, 2072–2076. [CrossRef]
13. Bamford, J.M.; Warlow, C.P. Evolution and testing of the lacunar hypothesis. *Stroke* **1988**, *19*, 1074–1082. [CrossRef] [PubMed]
14. Millikan, C.; Futrell, N. The fallacy of the lacune hypothesis. *Stroke* **1990**, *21*, 1251–1257. [CrossRef] [PubMed]
15. Gan, R.; Sacco, R.L.; Kargman, D.E.; Roberts, J.K.; Boden-Albala, B.; Gu, Q. Testing the validity of the lacunar hypothesis: The Northern Manhattan Stroke Study experience. *Neurology* **1997**, *48*, 1204–1211. [CrossRef] [PubMed]
16. Futrell, N. Lacunar infarction: Embolism is the key. *Stroke* **2004**, *35*, 1778–1779. [CrossRef] [PubMed]
17. Macdonald, R.L.; Kowalczuk, A.; Johns, L. Emboli enter penetrating arteries of monkey brain in relation to their size. *Stroke* **1995**, *26*, 1247–1250. [CrossRef] [PubMed]
18. Barnett, H.J.M.; Taylor, D.W.; Haynes, R.B.; Sackett, D.L.; Peerless, S.J.; Ferguson, G.G.; Fox, A.J.; Rankin, R.N.; Hachinski, V.C.; Wiebers, D.O.; et al. Beneficial effect of carotid endarterectomy in symptomatic patients with high-grade carotid stenosis. *N. Engl. J. Med.* **1991**, *325*, 445–453. [CrossRef]
19. Fisher, C.M.; Caplan, L.R. Basilar artery branch occlusion: A cause of pontine infarction. *Neurology* **1971**, *21*, 900–905. [CrossRef]
20. Fisher, C.M. Bilateral occlusion of basilar artery branches. *J. Neurol. Neurosurg. Psychiatry* **1977**, *40*, 1182–1189. [CrossRef]
21. Caplan, L.R. Intracranial branch atheromatous disease: A neglected, understudied, and underused concept. *Neurology* **1989**, *39*, 1246–1250. [CrossRef]
22. Jouvent, E.; Chabriat, H. Conventional imaging of lacunar infarcts. In *Cerebral Small Vessel Disease*; Pantoni, L., Gorelick, P.B., Eds.; Cambridge University Press: Cambridge, UK, 2014; pp. 129–138, ISBN 9781139382694.
23. Donnan, G.A.; Tress, B.M.; Bladin, P.F. A prospective study of lacunar infarction using computerized tomography. *Neurology* **1982**, *32*, 49–56. [CrossRef]
24. Nelson, R.F.; Pullicino, P.; Kendall, B.E.; Marshall, J. Computed tomography in patients presenting with lacunar syndromes. *Stroke* **1980**, *11*, 256–261. [CrossRef] [PubMed]
25. Alcalá, H.; Gado, M.; Torack, R.M. The effect of size, histologic elements, and water content on the visualization of cerebral infarcts. *Arch. Neurol.* **1978**, *35*, 1–7. [CrossRef] [PubMed]
26. Rascol, A.; Clanet, M.; Manelfe, C.; Guiraud, B.; Bonafe, A. Pure motor hemiplegia: CT study of 30 cases. *Stroke* **1982**, *13*, 11–17. [CrossRef] [PubMed]
27. Huang, C.; Woo, E.; Yu, Y.; Chan, F. Lacunar syndromes due to brainstem infarct and haemorrhage. *J. Neurol. Neurosurg. Psychiatry* **1988**, *51*, 509–515. [CrossRef]
28. Donnan, G.A.; Norrving, B. Chapter 27—Lacunes and lacunar syndromes. In *Handbook of Clinical Neurology*; Fisher, M., Ed.; Elsevier: Amsterdam, The Netherlands, 2008; Volume 93, pp. 559–575, ISBN 9780444520043.
29. Rothrock, J.F.; Lyden, P.D.; Hesselink, J.R.; Brown, J.J.; Healy, M.E. Brain magnetic resonance imaging in the evaluation of lacunar stroke. *Stroke* **1987**, *18*, 781–786. [CrossRef]

30. Brown, J.J.; Hesselink, J.R.; Rothrock, J.F. MR and CT of lacunar infarcts. *AJR. Am. J. Roentgenol.* **1988**, *151*, 367–372. [CrossRef]
31. Van Everdingen, K.J.; Van Der Grond, J.; Kappelle, L.J.; Ramos, L.M.P.; Mali, W.P.T.M. Diffusion-weighted magnetic resonance imaging in acute stroke. *Stroke* **1998**, *29*, 1783–1790. [CrossRef]
32. Wardlaw, J.M.; Smith, E.E.; Biessels, G.J.; Cordonnier, C.; Fazekas, F.; Frayne, R.; Lindley, R.I.; O'Brien, J.T.; Barkhof, F.; Benavente, O.R.; et al. Neuroimaging standards for research into small vessel disease and its contribution to ageing and neurodegeneration. *Lancet. Neurol.* **2013**, *12*, 822–838. [CrossRef]

© 2023 by the authors. Licensee MDPI, Basel, Switzerland. This article is an open access article distributed under the terms and conditions of the Creative Commons Attribution (CC BY) license (http://creativecommons.org/licenses/by/4.0/).

History of Vascular Cognitive Impairment and Dementia

Lukas Sveikata and Frédéric Assal

Abstract: Over the years, the definition of vascular cognitive impairment and dementia (VCID) has become a "moving target" due to demographic changes, advancements in the management of vascular risk factors, and neuroimaging. Since Sir Thomas Willis described the anatomy of brain blood supply (1664), "cerebral congestion" has become the main cause of dementia for several centuries. Later, the spotlight was on hypertensive arteriopathy, but as the population aged and hypertension management improved, the focus shifted to cerebral amyloid angiopathy and its contributions to dementia. The seminal pathological descriptions in the 1900s by Alzheimer and Binswanger put cerebrovascular disease on the map as one of the main drivers of cognitive dysfunction under the umbrella term of arteriosclerosis. It was not until the 1970s, with the advent of modern brain imaging, that the concept of vascular dementia (VaD) became widely accepted. The term VCID, on the other hand, was a result of developments in the understanding of a broad clinical spectrum of vascular disease, ranging from minor to major cognitive decline. The imaging revolution has led to the phenotyping of small-vessel disease, including the in vivo diagnosis of cerebral amyloid angiopathy, a key driver of VCID. Cerebrovascular disease has become widely recognized as the second most common form of dementia. In recent decades, the incidence of dementia was decreasing, leading to the recognition of vascular health as a major factor in brain health. We provide an overview of the field's evolution, from Sir Thomas Willis to our current understanding of VCID.

1. 17th to 19th Century—Apoplexy or the Concept of "Cerebral Congestion"

In the 17th century, stroke, referred to as the most typical form of apoplexy (from ancient Greek, "striking away"), was attributed to "cerebral congestion". Therefore, bloodletting was a common therapy until the introduction of the sphygmomanometer by Riva-Roci (1896) and Korotkov (1905) and the recognition of arterial hypertension as the primary cause of stroke.

The descriptions of Sir Thomas Willis (1621–1675) trace the origins of vascular dementia (VaD). In his work *De Anima Brutorum* [1], Willis wrote about his first case series of post-stroke dementia, describing the spectrum of clinical presentations from "dullness of mind and forgetfulness" to "stupidity and foolishness" accompanied by hemiplegia. He was also the first to recognize the ischemic nature of apoplexy. In *Cerebri Anatome* (1662) [2] he described an occlusion of the carotid artery and persistent collateral brain circulation —"The nature had substituted a sufficient remedy against the danger of Apoplexy", referring to the principal brain supplying arteries forming an anastomotic circle, named after him (Figure 1). Etienne Esquirol

(1772–1840) provided an anatomo-pathological report on 232 cases, identifying apoplexy as a potential cause of dementia [3]. Amédée Dechambre (1812–1886), a French physician, was the first to characterize "lacunes" (1838) in stroke survivors as small "cerebral softenings" (*ramollissement cérébral*) [4]. Five years later, Maxime Durand-Fardel (1843), the father of gerontology in France, independently postulated the pathogenesis of lacunes [5]. In 1854, Durand-Fardel described interstitial atrophy of the brain (compatible with modern-day *leukoaraiosis*) and *état criblé* (cribriform state, sieve-like state) reflecting chronic "cerebral congestion" [6].

In 1878, William Alexander Hammond (1828–1900), an American military physician and neurologist, stated the following:

> *Cerebral congestion is more common ... than any other affection of the nervous system ... the result of mental strain or emotional disturbance ... an outgrowth of our civilization, and of the restless spirit of enterprise and struggle for wealth ...* [7]

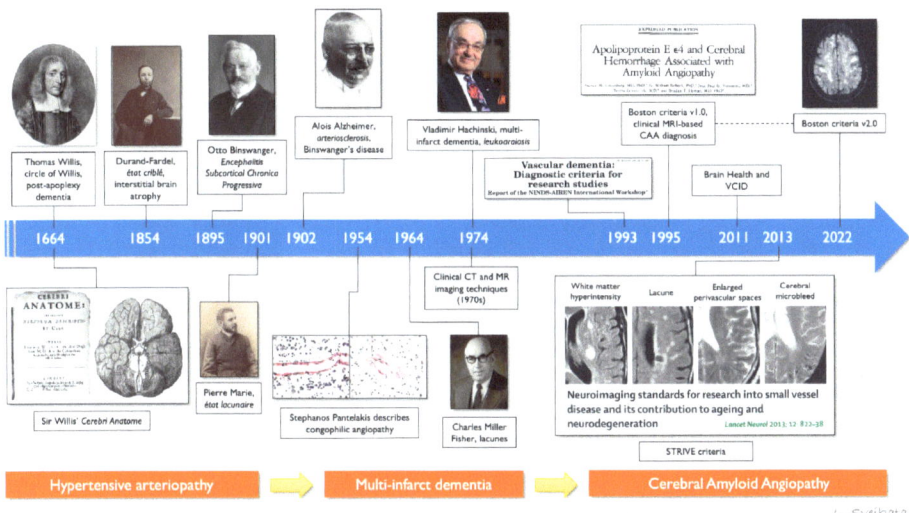

Figure 1. Principal clinician–scientists, their contributions, and major developments in vascular cognitive impairment and dementia (VCID). Over time, the field's focus has shifted from hypertensive arteriopathy to cerebral amyloid angiopathy as the primary pathology of interest, driven by population aging and better care for vascular risk factors. Source: Adapted from personal collection (V.H.) as well as Wardlaw et al. 2013 Lancet Neurol and Charidimou et al. 2022 Lancet Neurol, with permission from Elsevier.

2. 20th Century—Arteriosclerosis Confusion and the Dawn of Vascular Dementia

The modern history of VaD starts with Otto Binswanger (1852–1929) and Alois Alzheimer (1864–1915). The latter characterized arteriosclerotic brain atrophy (*arteriosclerotische Hirnatrophie*) and separated it from neurosyphilitic progressive paralysis (Table 1) [8]. In 1902, Alzheimer coined the name Binswanger's disease after the latter's description of white matter pallor as well as atrophy in one of his demented patients:

> *The disease has an insidious onset, with mild tiredness, headache, dizziness, decrease in sleep, followed by severe irritability and memory deficit. Alternatively, sudden onset with an apoplectiform attack and one-sided paralysis could initiate the picture.* [9]

Table 1. Historical terms used to describe vascular cognitive impairment and dementia. Source: Authors' compilation based on references provided in the table. Abbreviations: AHA/ASA, American Heart Association, American Stroke Association; AIREN, Association Internationale pour la Recherche et l'Enseignement en Neuroscience, NINDS, Neuroepidemiology Branch of the National Institute of Neurological Disorders and Stroke.

Term	Main Reference
Cerebral congestion	17th century
Post-apoplexy dementia	Thomas Willis (1672) [1]
Cerebral softenings (*ramollissement cérébral*), lacunes	Amédée Dechambre (1838) [4] and Durand-Fardel (1843) [5]
Interstitial brain atrophy and *etat criblé*	Durand-Fardel (1843) [5]
General arthritic pseudoparalysis (Klippel's disease)	Maurice Klippel (1892) [10]
Chronic progressive subcortical encephalopathy (*Encephalitis subcorticalis chronica progressiva*)	Otto Binswanger (1894) [11]
Arteriosclerotic dementia	Alois Alzheimer (1897) [12]
Etat lacunaire et criblé	Pierre Marie (1901) [13]
Binswanger's disease	Alois Alzheimer (1902) [9]
Senile dementia, arteriosclerosis	Emil Kraepelin (1910) [14]
Multi-infarct dementia	Vladimir Hachinski et al. (1974) [15]
Leukoaraiosis	Vladimir Hachinski et al. (1987) [16]
Vascular dementia	Gustavo Román et al. NINDS-AIREN criteria (1993) [17]
Vascular leukoencephalopathy	Unknown, but mostly derived from older CADASIL literature [18]
Subcortical ischemic vascular dementia	Gustavo Román et al. (2002) [19]
Post-stroke dementia	Didier Leys et al. (2005) [20]
Vascular cognitive impairment and dementia	Philip Gorelick et al. AHA/ASA Scientific Statement (2011) [21]

Alzheimer wondered whether white matter changes might be the result of secondary degeneration due to small infarcts, but he did not offer clear proof. He distinguished four clinicopathological variants of VaD: dementia post-apoplexy (later known as post-stroke dementia), arteriosclerotic brain degeneration (*état lacunaire* or *criblé*), senile cortical atrophy (granular atrophy), and subcortical encephalopathy (Binswanger's disease, later known as small-vessel disease). Interestingly, in the more severe forms of progressive arteriosclerotic brain degeneration, Alzheimer described multiple bleedings and softenings in the cerebral cortex as well as hemispheric white matter, possibly corresponding to microbleeds related to cerebral autosomal dominant arteriopathy with subcortical infarcts and leukoencephalopathy (CADASIL) or cerebral amyloid angiopathy (CAA).

Stephanos Pantelakis, a neuropathologist from Geneva Brain Collection, provided one of the first detailed pathological descriptions of congophilic angiopathy in 1954, known as modern-day CAA [22,23]. Subsequent studies supported Pantelakis' original discoveries that CAA impacts cortical and leptomeningeal vessels, that it was associated with age, dementia, its predilection for occipital lobes, and its absence of relation to arteriosclerosis. These findings paved the way for CAA as a unique disease entity, although it remained a pathological entity for several decades until its clinical manifestations of brain hemorrhaging and cognitive decline were attributed to the disease at the turn of the 21st century.

In the decades to come, Olszewski (1962) and Hachinski (1991) were skeptical of the existence of "so-called Binswanger's Disease" [24,25]. To them, Binswanger's description seemed to resemble leukodystrophies, Schilder's disease (currently a form of multiple sclerosis), or especially syphilitic changes. Notwithstanding, Binswanger also described two other forms of VaD: arteriosclerotic brain disease and dementia post-apoplexia, compatible with hypertensive arteriopathy and multi-infarct dementia, respectively [26]. One of the earliest illustrations of Binswanger's disease was published in the chapter on "Senile and Presenile Dementia" in the 1910 edition of Emil Kraepelin's seminal psychiatry textbook [14]. Kraepelin's influence was so prominent that, after the description of arteriosclerotic dementia and cerebral arteriosclerosis, the term "sclerosis" became synonymous with senile dementia for the next 70 years [27].

Pierre Marie (1853–1940), from the Hospice for the Elderly in Bicêtre, Paris, presented on *état lacunaire et criblé* at the 1901 congress in Paris [13]. For several decades there was some confusion between lacunes and *état criblé* until Charles Miller Fisher (1913–2012) published his landmark observations on lacunes in the 1960s [28,29]. He noted the frequent step-wise progression affecting speech, producing dysarthria, pseudobulbar signs, gait and instability problems, diplopia, aphasia, and confusion. He noted that "by the time the full course has been run, the patient may be immobilized by bilateral hemiparesis, incontinent, mute, and mindless" [30].

With the advent of neuroimaging, leukoaraiosis, derived from Greek root *leukos*, "white", and *araios*, "rarefied", was coined by Vladimir Hachinski and colleagues in 1987 [16]. The assumption of hypoperfusion causing vascular brain lesions led to decades of "blanket" treatment with vasodilation drugs, but all in vain [31]. Even upon detailed histopathological examination, Fisher did not observe vascular occlusions in penetrating arteries of the white matter, discarding the hypothesis that white matter disease was due to an occlusive mechanism [29,30]. Modern-era advanced neuroimaging techniques were also unable to demonstrate occlusion of a single artery leading to white matter injury [32].

3. End of the 20th and 21st Century: Neuroimaging Revolution

3.1. 1970s: From Multi-Infarct Dementia to VaD Subtypes

The advent of CT and, later, MRI imaging allowed for the in vivo identification of vascular contributions to dementia. In 1968, Charles Miller Fisher provided a lucid description of vascular dementia from his extensive experience, summarizing that "it is a matter of strokes large and small" [33]. The old and confusing term cerebral arteriosclerosis was replaced by multi-infarct dementia by Hachinski and colleagues in 1974 [15]. The latter concept was based on the mechanism that multiple brain infarcts of varying sizes ultimately cause cognitive deterioration. Although multi-infarct dementia and tools, such as the ischemic score, suggested a person's cerebrovascular burden, neither a causal nor temporal relation between vascular lesions and dementia was established [34].

A standardized diagnostic approach was required to advance the VaD field. The ADDTC criteria unified clinical and imaging criteria exclusively for ischemic VaD, requiring one or two strokes and a clear temporal relationship between a stroke and dementia onset [35]. DSM-IV and ICD-10 criteria were less restrictive but did not specify neuroimaging standards. VaD was recognized to have a much broader clinical spectrum than multi-infarct dementia under the 1993 NINDS-AIREN criteria, which included a subtype due to small-vessel disease [17]. Later, to emphasize the need for early detection and prevention, the term mild cognitive impairment of vascular origin or vascular cognitive impairment (VCI)—no dementia was proposed [36]. Next, because of relatively intact memory in VCI (relatively preserved integrity of mesial temporal lobes and thalami), the 2011 AHA/ASA criteria no longer required memory impairment to diagnose vascular dementia. The concept of brain health was also introduced [21]. The most recent VICCCS guidelines provided standardization of the VCI diagnosis based on MRI imaging, neuropsychological testing, and clinical components [37]. They encompassed a broad clinical spectrum, from mild to major VCI, and acknowledged subtypes of VCI, including mixed pathologies.

MRI became the gold standard and allowed for better phenotyping of small-vessel [38]. The delineation of ischemic and hemorrhagic imaging markers became possible. Iron-sensitive imaging allowed for the clinical identification of

CAA [39]. This was clinically relevant, as CAA was increasingly recognized as being highly prevalent in older adults. Importantly, combined vascular and AD pathologies lead to a higher likelihood of dementia than either pathology alone [40,41]. The most recent update of the Boston criteria v2.0, incorporated non-hemorrhagic imaging markers and improved diagnostic accuracy across a spectrum of clinical settings, including cognitive impairment without previous hemorrhage [42].

3.2. Diffuse White Matter Disease

Ischemic brain injury, commonly detected in pathology as macro- or microinfarcts related to small-vessel disease, was increasingly recognized as a driver of cognitive decline. Leveraging the arrival of MRI, Franz Fazekas and colleagues unified the WMH grading system in 1984 [43]. Later, Wahlund and colleagues developed a widely used clinical scale to rate age-related white matter changes [44]. In 2013, the STRIVE guidelines brought standardization to small-vessel disease imaging and terminology and, thus, made a significant advancement in the field [18]. White matter hyperintensities (WMHs) were proposed as an umbrella term to encompass different terms previously used to describe white matter changes, e.g., vascular leukoencephalopathy, Binswanger's disease, leukoaraiosis, etc. The WMHs term had a major advantage in terms of being purely descriptive and not attempting to delineate underlying tissue alteration mechanisms, as they are now known to be highly variable.

3.3. Mechanisms of Vascular Pathology

In recent decades, diffusion-weighted imaging has made it possible to recognize microinfarcts that despite their small size have significant effects on cognitive decline [45]. Microinfarcts became a marker of widespread vascular damage leading to disconnection syndrome [46]. As the underlying cellular function was better understood, the concepts of the blood–brain barrier [47] and neurovascular unit dysfunction [48] came to light.

The discovery of the NOTCH 3 gene related to CADASIL in 1996 greatly advanced research and understanding of the pathophysiology of small-vessel disease [49]. The discovery improved our understanding of the clinical and radiologic manifestations of "pure" vascular disease, independent of Alzheimer's disease [50].

Multiple neuropathological effects of the apolipoprotein E (ApoE) e4 allele have been identified, including decreased amyloid clearance, the loss of cerebrovascular integrity, and blood–brain barrier disintegration. In 1995, Greenberg and colleagues discovered that the presence of the ApoE ε4 allele raises the levels of both plaque and vascular amyloid, suggesting major implications for VCID [51]. Adults who were more likely to develop AD or CAA were able to be identified thanks to APOE genotyping. Contrarily, ApoE ε2 was found to be protective in AD but a risk factor for hemorrhagic CAA (for a review of this, see Greenberg et al. 2020 [52]).

4. Conclusions

The history of VCID starts with Sir Thomas Willis' description of post-apoplexy dementia, described as "dullness of mind and forgetfulness". In the two centuries that followed, the initial approach was focused on "brain congestion" and bloodletting. Over the years, the definition of VCID has become a "moving target" and shifted due to changes in population demography, improving vascular risk factor control, and advancement in neuroimaging. The vascular alterations in patients with dementia have been extensively discussed in seminal works by Alzheimer and Binswanger; however, the concepts of senile dementia (akin to Alzheimer's disease) and arteriosclerotic disease were used interchangeably for several decades. In the modern era, a subclassification of vascular dementia subtypes arose. This was followed by the concepts of vascular cognitive impairment and dementia, which were more inclusive and encompassed both ischemic and hemorrhagic vascular brain alterations. The identification of small-vessel disease, including CAA in vivo, expanded the boundaries of our knowledge of the linkages between vascular and Alzheimer's disease. As a result of better blood pressure control and improved vascular health, the incidence of dementia has been declining in recent years [44]. This intriguing finding suggests that vascular dementia may be the most curable and, possibly, most fascinating type of dementia. The evolution of VCID has proven once again that "The problems are immense, but the opportunities are even greater" [53].

Author Contributions: L.S. drafted the manuscript, while both authors revised and approved the published version. All authors have read and agreed to the published version of the manuscript.

Funding: Lukas Sveikata was supported by the Swiss National Science Foundation postdoctoral award (P2GEP3_191584). Frédéric Assal was supported by the FNS Sinergia CRSII5_202228, FNS 4078P0_198438/1].

Acknowledgments: We thank Andreas Charidimou for his critical review and suggestions to the manuscript. The figure elements were reproduced with permission from Vladimir Hachinski and Elsevier.

Conflicts of Interest: The authors have no conflicts of interest to declare.

References

1. Willis, T. *De anima brutorum*; Davis: London, UK, 1672.
2. Willis, T. *Cerebri anatome: Cui accessit nervorum descriptio et usus*; Martin & Allestry by University College London: London, UK, 1664.
3. Esquirol, E. *Des Maladies Mentales Considérées Sous les Rapports Médical, Hygiénique et Médico-Légal*; J.-B. Baillière: Paris, France, 1938.
4. Dechambre, A. Mémoire sur la curabilité du ramollissement cérébral. *Gazette Medicale de Paris* **1838**, *6*, 305–314.
5. Durand-Fardel, M. *Traité du ramollissement du cerveau*; J.-B. Baillière: Paris, France, 1843.
6. Durand-Fardel, M. *Traité clinique et pratique des maladies des vieillards*; G. Baillière: Paris, France, 1854.

7. Hammond, W.A. *Cerebral Hyperæmia; The Result of Mental Strain or Emotional Disturbance*; G.P. Putnam's Sons: New York, NY, USA, 1879.
8. Alzheimer, A. Die arteriosklerotische atrophie des gehirns. *Neurol Cent.* **1894**, *51*, 1809–1812.
9. Alzheimer, A. Die Seelenstörungen auf arteriosclerotischer Grundlage. *Allg. Z Psychiatr. Psych.-Gerichtl. Med.* **1902**, *59*, 695–711.
10. Klippel, M. De la pseudoparalysie générale arthritique. *Rev. De Méd.* **1892**, *12*, 280–285.
11. Binswanger, O. Die Abgrenzung der allgemeinen progressiven Paralyse. *Berl. Klin Wochenschr.* **1894**, *49*, 1103–1105, 1137–1139, 1180–1186.
12. Alzheimer, A. Ueber perivasculaere Gliose. *Allg. Z Psychiatr. Psych. Med.* **1897**, *53*, 863–865.
13. Marie, P. Des foyers lacunaires de désintégration et de différents autres états cavitaires du cerveau. *Rev. Méd.* **1901**, *21*, 281–298.
14. Kraepelin, E. *Psychiatrie. Ein Lehrbuch für Studierende und Ärzte. II. Band*; Johann Ambrosius Barth: Leipzig, Germany, 1910.
15. Hachinski, V.C.; Lassen, N.A.; Marshall, J. Multi-infarct dementia a cause of mental deterioration in the elderly. *Lancet* **1974**, *304*, 207–209. [CrossRef]
16. Hachinski, V.C.; Potter, P.; Merskey, H. Leuko-Araiosis. *Arch. Neurol.-Chic.* **1987**, *44*, 21–23. [CrossRef]
17. Roman, G.C.; Tatemichi, T.K.; Erkinjuntti, T.; Cummings, J.L.; Masdeu, J.C.; Garcia, J.H.; Amaducci, L.; Orgogozo, J.-M.; Brun, A.; Hofman, A.; et al. Vascular dementia: Diagnostic criteria for research studies: Report of the NINDS-AIREN International Workshop. *Neurology* **1993**, *43*, 250. [CrossRef]
18. Wardlaw, J.M.; Smith, E.E.; Biessels, G.J.; Cordonnier, C.; Fazekas, F.; Frayne, R.; Lindley, R.I.; O'Brien, J.T.; Barkhof, F.; Benavente, O.R.; et al. Neuroimaging standards for research into small vessel disease and its contribution to ageing and neurodegeneration. *Lancet Neurol.* **2013**, *12*, 822–838. [CrossRef] [PubMed]
19. Román, G.C.; Erkinjuntti, T.; Wallin, A.; Pantoni, L.; Chui, H.C. Subcortical ischaemic vascular dementia. *Lancet Neurol.* **2002**, *1*, 426–436. [CrossRef] [PubMed]
20. Leys, D.; Hénon, H.; Mackowiak-Cordoliani, M.-A.; Pasquier, F. Poststroke dementia. *Lancet Neurol.* **2005**, *4*, 752–759. [CrossRef]
21. Gorelick, P.B.; Scuteri, A.; Black, S.E.; DeCarli, C.; Greenberg, S.M.; Iadecola, C.; Launer, L.J.; Laurent, S.; Lopez, O.L.; Nyenhuis, D.; et al. Vascular Contributions to Cognitive Impairment and Dementia. *Stroke* **2011**, *42*, 2672–2713. [CrossRef] [PubMed]
22. Kövari, E.; Hof, P.R.; Bouras, C. The Geneva brain collection. *Ann. N. Y. Acad. Sci.* **2011**, *1225*, E131–E146. [CrossRef]
23. Pantelakis, S. Un type particulier d'angiopathie sénile du système nerveux central: L'angiopathie congophile. Topographie et fréquence; pp. 219–237. *Eur. Neurol.* **1954**, *128*, 219–237. [CrossRef]
24. Hachinski, V. Binswanger's disease: Neither Binswanger's nor a disease. *J. Neurol. Sci.* **1991**, *103*, 1. [CrossRef]
25. Olszewski, J. Subcortical arteriosclerotic encephalopathy. Review of the literature on the so-called Binswanger's disease and presentation of two cases. *World Neurol.* **1962**, *3*, 359–375.

26. Mast, H.; Tatemichi, T.K.; Mohr, J.P. Chronic brain ischemia: The contributions of Otto Binswanger and Alois Alzheimer to the mechanisms of vascular dementia. *J. Neurol. Sci.* **1995**, *132*, 4–10. [CrossRef]
27. Román, G. Vascular Dementia: A Historical Background. *Int. Psychogeriatr.* **2003**, *15*, 11–13. [CrossRef]
28. Fisher, C.M. Lacunes Small, deep cerebral infarcts. *Neurology* **1965**, *15*, 774. [CrossRef] [PubMed]
29. Fisher, C.M. The arterial lesions underlying lacunes. *Acta Neuropathol.* **1969**, *12*, 1–15. [CrossRef] [PubMed]
30. Fisher, C.M. Binswanger's encephalopathy: A review. *J. Neurol.* **1989**, *236*, 65–79. [CrossRef] [PubMed]
31. Frackowiak, R.S.J.; Pozzilli, C.; Legg, N.J.; Boulay, G.H.; Marshall, J.; Lenzi, G.L.; Jones, T. Regional cerebral oxygen supply and utilization in dementia: A clinical and physiological study with oxygen-15 and positron tomography a clinical and physiological study with oxygen-15 and positron tomography. *Brain* **1981**, *104*, 753–778. [CrossRef] [PubMed]
32. Wardlaw, J.M.; Dennis, M.S.; Warlow, C.P.; Sandercock, P.A. Imaging appearance of the symptomatic perforating artery in patients with lacunar infarction: Occlusion or other vascular pathology? *Ann. Neurol.* **2001**, *50*, 208–215. [CrossRef] [PubMed]
33. Fisher, C.M. Dementia in cerebral vascular disease. In *Cerebral Vascular Diseases: Sixth Princeton Conference*; Toole, J.F., Siekert, R.G., Whisnant, J.P., Eds.; Grune & Stratton: New York, NY, USA, 1968; pp. 232–236.
34. Hachinski, V.C.; Iliff, L.D.; Zilhka, E.; Boulay, G.H.D.; McAllister, V.L.; Marshall, J.; Russell, R.W.R.; Symon, L. Cerebral Blood Flow in Dementia. *Arch. Neurol.-Chic.* **1975**, *32*, 632–637. [CrossRef]
35. Chui, H.C.; Victoroff, J.I.; Margolin, D.; Jagust, W.; Shankle, R.; Katzman, R. Criteria for the diagnosis of ischemic vascular dementia proposed by the State of California Alzheimer's Disease Diagnostic and Treatment Centers. *Neurology* **1992**, *42*, 473. [CrossRef]
36. Bowler, J.; Hachinski, V. Vascular cognitive impairment: A new approach to vascular dementia. In *Bailliere's Clinical Neurology*; Elsevier: Amsterdam, The Netherlands, 1995; Volume 4, pp. 357–376.
37. Skrobot, O.A.; Black, S.E.; Chen, C.; DeCarli, C.; Erkinjuntti, T.; Ford, G.A.; Kalaria, R.N.; O'Brien, J.; Pantoni, L.; Pasquier, F.; et al. Progress toward standardized diagnosis of vascular cognitive impairment: Guidelines from the Vascular Impairment of Cognition Classification Consensus Study. *Alzheimer's Dement.* **2018**, *14*, 280–292. [CrossRef]
38. Zotin, M.C.Z.; Sveikata, L.; Viswanathan, A.; Yilmaz, P. Cerebral small vessel disease and vascular cognitive impairment: From diagnosis to management. *Curr. Opin. Neurol.* **2021**, *34*, 246–257. [CrossRef]
39. Greenberg, S.M.; Vonsattel, J.P.G.; Stakes, J.W.; Gruber, M.; Finklestein, S.P. The clinical spectrum of cerebral amyloid angiopathy: Presentations without lobar hemorrhage. *Neurology* **1993**, *43*, 2073. [CrossRef]
40. Viswanathan, A.; Greenberg, S.M. Cerebral amyloid angiopathy in the elderly. *Ann. Neurol.* **2011**, *70*, 871–880. [CrossRef] [PubMed]

41. Zekry, D.; Duyckaerts, C.; Moulias, R.; Belmin, J.; Geoffre, C.; Herrmann, F.; Hauw, J.-J. Degenerative and vascular lesions of the brain have synergistic effects in dementia of the elderly. *Acta Neuropathol.* **2002**, *103*, 481–487. [CrossRef] [PubMed]
42. Charidimou, A.; Boulouis, G.; Frosch, M.P.; Baron, J.-C.; Pasi, M.; Albucher, J.F.; Banerjee, G.; Barbato, C.; Bonneville, F.; Brandner, S.; et al. The Boston criteria version 2.0 for cerebral amyloid angiopathy: A multicentre, retrospective, MRI–neuropathology diagnostic accuracy study. *Lancet Neurol.* **2022**, *21*, 714–725. [CrossRef] [PubMed]
43. Fazekas, F.; Chawluk, J.; Alavi, A.; Hurtig, H.; Zimmerman, R. MR signal abnormalities at 1.5 T in Alzheimer's dementia and normal aging. *Am. J. Roentgenol.* **1987**, *149*, 351–356. [CrossRef]
44. Wahlund, L.O.; Barkhof, F.; Fazekas, F.; Bronge, L.; Augustin, M.; Sjögren, M.; Wallin, A.; Ader, H.; Leys, D.; Pantoni, L.; et al. A New Rating Scale for Age-Related White Matter Changes Applicable to MRI and CT. *Stroke* **2001**, *32*, 1318–1322. [CrossRef]
45. Van Veluw, S.J.; Shih, A.Y.; Smith, E.E.; Chen, C.; Schneider, J.A.; Wardlaw, J.M.; Greenberg, S.M.; Biessels, G.J. Detection, risk factors, and functional consequences of cerebral microinfarcts. *Lancet Neurol.* **2017**, *16*, 730–740. [CrossRef]
46. Ter Telgte, A.; van Leijsen, E.M.C.; Wiegertjes, K.; Klijn, C.J.M.; Tuladhar, A.M.; de Leeuw, F.-E. Cerebral small vessel disease: From a focal to a global perspective. *Nat. Rev. Neurol.* **2018**, *14*, 387–398. [CrossRef]
47. Wardlaw, J.M.; Sandercock, P.A.G.; Dennis, M.S.; Starr, J. Is Breakdown of the Blood-Brain Barrier Responsible for Lacunar Stroke, Leukoaraiosis, and Dementia? *Stroke J. Am. Heart Assoc.* **2003**, *34*, 806–812. [CrossRef]
48. Iadecola, C. The Neurovascular Unit Coming of Age: A Journey through Neurovascular Coupling in Health and Disease. *Neuron* **2017**, *96*, 17–42. [CrossRef]
49. Joutel, A.; Corpechot, C.; Ducros, A.; Vahedi, K.; Chabriat, H.; Mouton, P.; Alamowitch, S.; Domenga, V.; Cécillion, M.; Maréchal, E.; et al. Notch3 mutations in CADASIL, a hereditary adult-onset condition causing stroke and dementia. *Nature* **1996**, *383*, 707–710. [CrossRef]
50. Buffon, F.; Porcher, R.; Hernandez, K.; Kurtz, A.; Pointeau, S.; Vahedi, K.; Bousser, M.-G.; Chabriat, H. Cognitive profile in CADASIL. *J. Neurol. Neurosurg. Psychiatry* **2006**, *77*, 175. [CrossRef] [PubMed]
51. Greenberg, S.M.; Rebeck, G.W.; Vonsattel, J.P.G.; Gomez-Isla, T.; Hyman, B.T. Apolipoprotein E ε4 and cerebral hemorrhage associated with amyloid angiopathy. *Ann. Neurol.* **1995**, *38*, 254–259. [CrossRef] [PubMed]
52. Greenberg, S.M.; Bacskai, B.J.; Hernandez-Guillamon, M.; Pruzin, J.; Sperling, R.; van Veluw, S.J. Cerebral amyloid angiopathy and Alzheimer disease—One peptide, two pathways. *Nat. Rev. Neurol.* **2020**, *16*, 30–42. [CrossRef] [PubMed]
53. Hachinski, V. Vascular Dementia: A Radical Redefinition. *Dement. Geriatr. Cogn.* **1994**, *5*, 130–132. [CrossRef] [PubMed]

© 2023 by the authors. Licensee MDPI, Basel, Switzerland. This article is an open access article distributed under the terms and conditions of the Creative Commons Attribution (CC BY) license (http://creativecommons.org/licenses/by/4.0/).

Part III: Progress in Diagnosis and Treatment: The Last 50 Years

Progress in Diagnosis and Treatment: The Last 50 Years of Stroke Prevention

Kateryna Antonenko and Maria Giulia Mosconi

Abstract: Stroke is a major global health issue. However, up to 85% of strokes may be preventable. Following an integrated conceptual timeline, we briefly report historical notes on the birth of and advancements in research on the pathophysiology and treatments of the major risk factors associated with ischemic stroke. We finally focused on the last 50 years, representing a landmark in the progress of stroke medicine. We reviewed and reported the results of the significant trials on the main stroke risk factors. The design and the results of large-scale epidemiological studies have clarified many of the underlying mechanisms of stroke pathophysiology, which has led to impressive developments in treating diseases that were considered untreatable for centuries. Although stroke is a largely preventable disease, there are still many issues faced when implementing strategies to reduce the global burden of the disease, both in terms of primary and secondary prevention.

1. Introduction

Stroke remains a major global health problem. However, up to 85% of strokes may be preventable [1]. Primary and secondary stroke prevention has significantly evolved in the last half-century, moving to the forefront of stroke management strategies. Ten potentially modifiable risk factors cause 90% of all strokes, and the most transparent approach to reducing the stroke burden is to target these factors using novel practical approaches. The World Health Organization states that effective stroke prevention tactics include decreasing the risk associated with systemic blood hypertension, diabetes mellitus, dyslipidemia, a non-healthy diet, a sedentary lifestyle, smoking, and abdominal obesity [2]. Considering the historical aspects of the last 50 years, it is interesting that the first prospective multicenter randomized trials and first advances in stroke care appeared earlier in stroke prevention than in stroke treatment.

2. Literature Review

We briefly reported the history on the birth of and advancements in research on the pathophysiology and treatments of the major risk factors associated with ischemic stroke.

We finally focused on the last 50 years, representing a landmark in progress in stroke medicine.

We reviewed and reported the results of the significant trials on the main stroke risk factors, searching PubMed and MEDLINE.

2.1. Antiplatelets

Synthetic aspirin is derived from salicylic acid, a natural compound from myrtle, willow, and meadowsweet, which has been used in herbal medicine since ancient times for its anti-inflammatory effects. Clay tablets from the Assyrians (around 2000 BCE) showcase that willow leaves were advised for the treatment of rheumatic disease; moreover, Hippocrates (460–377 BCE) prescribed an extract of willow bark for labor and fever pain [3]. In 1876, Dr. T. MacLagan performed the first clinical study of salicylate by administering salicin to achieve the full remission of joint inflammation and fever in patients suffering from acute rheumatism. In 1897, Dr. F. Hoffman produced pure, stable acetylsalicylic acid (ASA), thus creating both aspirin and the pharmaceutical manufacturing industry. On 1 February 1899, the new substance was named and first registered as aspirin [4].

We have to wait until 1953, when Dr. Craven first suggested the role of aspirin as an antithrombotic drug, publishing his work on the prevention of coronary thrombosis [5].

Weiss and Aledort, in 1967, described the irreversible suppression determined by aspirin on platelet aggregation [6], and, four years later, Vane reported the inhibition of prostaglandin synthesis as an additional mechanism of the action of aspirin [7]. After Vane received the Nobel Prize for Medicine in 1982, aspirin became established as a drug for the treatment and prevention of cardiovascular diseases.

The first trials demonstrate successful stroke prevention by aspirin, combined with other drugs (e.g., dipyridamole, ticlopidine, and sulfinpyrazone), dating back to 1970–1980 [8,9]. The Antiplatelet Trialists' Collaboration reported in 1988 that aspirin reduced overall vascular death by 15% and the incidence of non-fatal stroke and myocardial infarction by 30% [10]; the same year, the US Food and Drug Administration (FDA) granted final approval of aspirin for ischemic stroke prevention in the United States. In 1996, a CAPRIE study reported the effectiveness of clopidogrel in stroke prevention [11]. Pooled analysis of CHANCE and POINT trials in 2019 showed the benefits of dual antiaggregant treatment with the association of clopidogrel and aspirin for the secondary prevention of minor ischemic stroke or high-risk transient ischemic attack (TIA) [12].

2.2. Anticoagulants

The first agent with anticoagulant activity was discovered in dog liver by McLean et al. in 1916., which would have been known as heparin [13]. Heparin purification and sufficient production for clinical use and the discovery of its dependency on a plasma factor (now known as antithrombin) for its anticoagulant action date back to the 1930s [14].

Oral anticoagulation has a dramatic story, starting in the 1920s with the discovery of dicoumarol when, in Canada, cattle began dying of internal bleeding without an identifiable triggering cause. F. W. Schofield, a veterinary pathologist, determined that the mysterious disease was related to the ingestion of spoiled sweet clover hay and reported a prolonged clotting time [15]. Oral anticoagulants were first designed in the 1930s and introduced for clinical use in 1959 when dicumarol was identified as the substance contained in moldy clover [16].

A series of randomized controlled trials (RCTs) on anticoagulation with warfarin, conducted in the late 1980s and early 1990s for primary and secondary stroke prevention, reported a significant reduction in the rate of ischemic stroke in patients affected by atrial fibrillation [17]. In 1997, the IST results reported that early anticoagulation with unfractionated heparin reduced recurrent ischemic stroke but significantly increased hemorrhagic stroke, without a net decrease in recurrent stroke, death, or dependency [18]. An adjusted warfarin dose (international normalized ratio range between 2.0 and 3.0) and antiplatelet therapy have been shown to decrease stroke risk by approximately two-thirds and one-fifth, respectively, in comparison to the controls [19], but not in patients with sinus rhythm [20].

Since 2009, four large RCTs have reported the non-inferiority of four direct oral anticoagulants (DOACs) over adjusted-dose warfarin for stroke prophylaxis in non-valvular atrial fibrillation (NVAF), with a favorable risk–benefit profile [21–25]. Currently, DOACs are recommended for both primary and secondary stroke prevention management in individuals suffering from NVAF.

Regarding clinical atherosclerotic disease, the results of a post hoc sub-analysis of the COMPASS trial [26] in patients with non-lacunar, non-cardioembolic ischemic stroke, along with clinical atherosclerotic disease, reported that low-dose (2.5 mg twice daily) therapy with rivaroxaban plus aspirin (100mg daily) may significantly reduce the rate of ischemic events for both primary and secondary stroke prevention [27].

New anticoagulant agents under investigation in phase 2 trials are the activated coagulation factor XI inhibitors. From phase I studies results, they are reported as being associated with lower bleeding rates. Recent PACIFIC AF study highlighted that, in patients with NVAF, the FXIa inhibitor asundexian reduced bleeding rates compared with standard dosing of apixaban, with near-complete in vivo FXIa inhibition [28].

2.3. Carotid Revascularization

After early failures in the 1940s–1950s in China [29] and Argentina [30], the first successful carotid endarterectomy was conducted in 1953 in the USA by M. DeBakey [31]. The first RCT of carotid endarterectomy was started in 1962, and its results reported benefits from the procedure but a high rate of complications [32]. In 1987, H. J. M. Barnett designed the NASCET trial [33], a large-scale clinical trial on patients with carotid disease symptomatic for TIAs or minor stroke, to estimate the risk–benefit ratio of carotid endarterectomy. In 1991, a net benefit of the surgical intervention in patients with a stenosis of the internal carotid artery greater than 70% was reported [33]. The same year, results obtained by the European ECST trial similarly showed the benefit of endarterecomy in comparison to medical management for patients with symptomatic severe carotid stenosis [34]. The rate of carotid endarterectomies, conducted for stroke prevention, following these results, has gradually increased over time [35].

2.4. Antihypertensive Treatment

The history of hypertension originates from ancient Chinese and Indian Ayurvedic medicine, where the quality of an individual's pulse, as palpated by the physician, was considered a gateway to the state of the cardiovascular system [36]. The modern concept of hypertension begins with the work of Dr. W. Harvey. He increased our understanding of the cardiovascular system, describing blood circulation in his text "De motu cordis" (1578–1657).

During the 18th century, the theory of blood pressure gradually gained acceptance. At the beginning of the 19th century, bloodletting evolved from a "means of restoring the balance of the humors" to a way of reducing blood pressure [37].

In the 20th century, particularly over the last 50 years, the medical community accepted that hypertension is a treatable disease and not an essential condition. Results from longitudinal studies, such as the "Framingham Heart Study" in 1974, highlighted that "benign" hypertension increased rates of death and cardiovascular disease. These risks increased proportionally with the increase in blood pressure values.

From 1967 to 2001, an increasing number of trials comparing the treatment of patients affected by moderate, then mild, diastolic and systolic hypertension with placebo (or routine care) demonstrated that lowering elevated blood pressure reduced the incidence of stroke, especially in primary prevention [35,38–42].

The PROGRESS trial in 2001 was the first large trial on the pharmacological management of hypertension in secondary stroke prevention [43]; the results showed that antihypertensive therapy with an angiotensin-converting enzyme inhibitor reduces the recurrence rate of stroke by 28% compared with placebo. Subsequently, since 2003, major international guidelines have recommended active treatment to lower blood pressure in patients with previous stroke [44–47].

Additionally, in 2014, AHA/ASA published the first set of guidelines on stroke prevention in women, reporting that there are several sex peculiarities in the pathophysiology, prevalence and therapy responses of hypertension that should be pointed to improve both the awareness and treatment of this risk factor in women [48].

2.5. Lipid-Lowering Drugs

Although commonly assumed to be a modern disease, atherosclerosis has been reported to be common in preindustrial, premodern human beings [49]. The association between atherosclerosis and lipids came much later. In 1833, cholesterol was first reported in human blood by F. H. Boudet, while in 1856, R. Virchow described atherosclerotic plaque as a fundamental lesion of atherosclerosis [50].

In 1932, Wieland reported the correct structure of cholesterol [51]. The link between lipoproteins and cardiovascular disorders backdates to the early 1950s [52]. Several drugs were investigated for their potential in reducing cholesterol plasma levels, before landing the breakthrough of statins in the 1970s: nicotinic acid, resins, fibrates.

In 1987, the first 3-hydroxy-3-methyl-glutaryl-CoA (HMG-CoA) reductase inhibitor for cholesterol reduction, lovastatin, was approved for clinical use by the US FDA, followed by simvastatin and pravastatin in 1989. By 2010, two semi-synthetic and four synthetic statins (e.g., simvastatin and pravastatin, in 1991; fluvastatin, 1994, atorvastatin, 1996, rosuvastatin, 2003, and pitavastatin, 2010) were marketed [53].

In 2006, the SPARCL trial reported the efficacy of high-dose statin therapy (80 mg atorvastatin daily) for secondary stroke prophylaxis [54]. Moreover, the "Treat Stroke to Target" trial results recently reported that patients in the lower target group (LDL target < 70 mg/dL) had a reduced risk of the composite primary endpoint of major cardiovascular events compared with patients in the higher target group (LDL target range: 90–110 mg/dL) in secondary stroke prevention [55].

In 2002, ezetimibe, an inhibitor of the intestinal absorption of cholesterol and other sterols, was introduced in clinical practice. The combination of ezetimibe plus statin has a synergistic mechanism, allowing the use of lower doses of statin, thereby minimizing their associated adverse effects [56]. In this regard, the 2019 European guidelines on dyslipidemia recommend the prescription of ezetimibe in patients who do not reach lipid targets with a statin alone [57].

In 2003, N. Seidah discovered proprotein convertase subtilisin Kexin-9 (PCSK-9), and its mutation was identified as a cause of autosomal dominant hypercholesterolemia. Alirocumab and evolocumab, wholly human anti-PCSK-9 antibodies, were accepted by the FDA [58] after their positive large trials results (FOURIER [59] and ODYSSEY [60]).

2.6. Antidiabetic Treatment

The mention of an illness characterized by the "too great emptying of urine" can be found in Egyptian manuscripts, more than 3000 years ago; moreover, Indian medicine reported it as madhumeha ("honey urine") because of its feature of attracting ants [61]. The first complete description of the disease is attributed to Aretaeus, the Cappadocian in the 1st century A.D., who conceived the word diabetes and affirmed, "No essential part of the drink is absorbed by the body while great masses of the flesh are liquefied into urine" [61]. The term mellitus was added by Dr. J. Rollo much later, in 1798, to distinguish this type from insipidus diabetes, with tasteless urine. The role of the pancreas in diabetes was described in 1889 by J. von Mering and O. Minkowski by showing that its removal renders dogs diabetic. Diet and exercise were the essentials of diabetes therapy in the 19th century [62]. Nobel prizes were awarded to J. J. R. Macleod and Sir F. G. Banting, in collaboration with C. H. Best, for isolating insulin and reporting the efficacious treatment of diabetic dogs by administering them pancreatic islets extract of healthy dogs. Insulin extract was finally purified by J. B. Collip for administration to humans; in 1922, Leonard Thompson, a 14-year-old boy, was the first patient to be successfully treated with insulin.

In 1948, H. Root first observed that hyperglycemia was linked to vascular disease. In 1993, this association was confirmed by the "Diabetes Control and Complications Trial" (DCCT) results [63].

The first oral medication for diabetes has been widespread since 1955, with the introduction of sulfonylureas [64].

Currently, diabetes is an undiscussed and impacting risk factor for stroke.

From early 2000, along with essential antidiabetic treatment, newer antidiabetic medications have become available: glucagon-like peptide-1 receptor (GLP-1R) agonists, sodium-glucose transport protein-2 inhibitors, and peroxisome proliferator-activated receptor-gamma agonists (PPAR-γ).

Among the GLP-1R agonists, preliminary data from the randomized REWIND trial showed that patients in the dulaglutide-treatment arm showed a significant reduction in ischemic stroke risk [65]. A 2020 systematic review and meta-analysis suggested that GLP-1R agonists significantly reduce incidents and non-fatal strokes [66].

In the case of insulin resistance, pioglitazone, a PPAR-γ agonist, demonstrated its efficacy for secondary stroke prevention. Secondary analysis of the IRIS trial reported that patients who suffered from an ischemic stroke or TIA, with no history of diabetes but affected by insulin resistance, if treated with pioglitazone, had a significant reduction in ischemic stroke rates when compared to placebo [67].

3. Conclusions

In the last 50 years, stroke medicine has undergone impressive advances thanks to new imaging techniques, stroke units' birth and spread, and revascularization therapies, making an "untreatable" disease curable.

Although it is widely acknowledged that stroke is a largely preventable disease [1], both in primary and secondary prophylaxis, taking into account the continuous development of pharmacological approaches and surgical, vascular procedures, there are still substantial gaps to achieving actions to reduce the global burden of the disease, notably in low–middle-income countries [68].

Author Contributions: K.A. and M.G.M equally contributed in conceptualization, methodology, review of the literature, in writing—original draft preparation, K.A. and M.G.M.; writing—review and editing. M.G.M.did the final uniformation of the contents presentation. All authors have read and agreed to the published version of the manuscript.

Funding: This research received no external funding.

Acknowledgments: We would like to thank Valeria Caso and Maurizio Paciaroni for their mentoring this paper.

Conflicts of Interest: The authors declare no conflict of interest.

References

1. O'Donnell, M.J.; Xavier, D.; Liu, L.; Zhang, H.; Chin, S.L.; Rao-Melacini, P.; Rangarajan, S.; Islam, S.; Pais, P.; McQueen, M.J.; et al. Risk factors for ischaemic and intracerebral haemorrhagic stroke in 22 countries (the INTERSTROKE study): A case-control study. *Lancet* **2010**, *376*, 112–123. [CrossRef]
2. Johnson, W.; Onuma, O.; Owolabi, M.; Sachdev, S. Stroke: A global response is needed. *Bull. World Health Organ.* **2016**, *94*, 634. [CrossRef]
3. Walker, J.; Hutchison, P.; Ge, J.; Zhao, D.; Wang, Y.; Rothwell, P.M.; Gaziano, J.M.; Chan, A.; Burn, J.; Chia, J.; et al. Aspirin: 120 years of innovation. A report from the 2017 Scientific Conference of the International Aspirin Foundation, 14 September 2017, Charité, Berlin. *Ecancermedicalscience* **2018**, *12*, 813. [CrossRef]
4. Jack, D.B. One hundred years of aspirin. *Lancet* **1997**, *350*, 437–439. [CrossRef]
5. Craven, L.L. Experiences with aspirin (Acetylsalicylic acid) in the nonspecific prophylaxis of coronary thrombosis. *Miss. Val. Med. J.* **1953**, *75*, 38–44.
6. Weiss, H.; Aledort, L. Impaired platelet/connective-tissue reaction in man after aspirin ingestion. *Lancet* **1967**, *290*, 495–497. [CrossRef] [PubMed]
7. Vane, J.R. Inhibition of Prostaglandin Synthesis as a Mechanism of Action for Aspirin-like Drugs. *Nat. New Biol.* **1971**, *231*, 232–235. [CrossRef] [PubMed]
8. Hass, W.K.; Easton, J.D.; Adams, H.P.; Pryse-Phillips, W.; Molony, B.A.; Anderson, S.; Kamm, B.; for the Ticlopidine Aspirin Stroke Study Group. A Randomized Trial Comparing Ticlopidine Hydrochloride with Aspirin for the Prevention of Stroke in High-Risk Patients. *N. Engl. J. Med.* **1989**, *321*, 501–507. [CrossRef]
9. Halkes, P.H.; Van Gijn, J.; Kappelle, L.J.; Koudstaal, P.J.; Algra, A. Aspirin plus dipyridamole versus aspirin alone after cerebral ischaemia of arterial origin (ESPRIT): Randomised controlled trial. *Lancet* **2006**, *367*, 1665–1673.
10. Antiplatelet Trialists' Collaboration. Secondary prevention of vascular disease by prolonged antiplatelet treatment. Antiplatelet Trialists' Collaboration. *Br. Med. J. (Clin. Res. Ed.)* **1988**, *296*, 320–331. [CrossRef]
11. Committee, C.S. A randomised, blinded, trial of clopidogrel versus aspirin in patients at risk of ischaemic events (CAPRIE). CAPRIE Steering Committee. *Lancet* **1996**, *348*, 1329–1339.
12. Pan, Y.; Elm, J.J.; Li, H.; Easton, J.D.; Wang, Y.; Farrant, M.; Meng, X.; Kim, A.S.; Zhao, X.; Meurer, W.J.; et al. Outcomes Associated with Clopidogrel-Aspirin Use in Minor Stroke or Transient Ischemic Attack: A Pooled Analysis of Clopidogrel in High-Risk Patients with Acute Non-Disabling Cerebrovascular Events (CHANCE) and Platelet-Oriented Inhibition in New TIA and Minor Ischemic Stroke (POINT) Trials. *JAMA Neurol.* **2019**, *76*, 1466–1473. [PubMed]
13. McLean, J. The Thromboplastic Action of Cephalin. *Am. J. Physiol.-Legacy Content* **1916**, *41*, 250–257. [CrossRef]
14. Barrowcliffe, T.W. History of heparin. *Handb. Exp. Pharmacol.* **2012**, 3–22.
15. Norn, S.; Permin, H.; Kruse, E.; Kruse, P.R. On the history of vitamin K, dicoumarol and warfarin. *Dan. Med. Arbog* **2014**, *42*, 99–119.
16. Link, K.P. The Discovery of Dicumarol and Its Sequels. *Circulation* **1959**, *19*, 97–107. [CrossRef] [PubMed]

17. Atrial Fibrillation Investigators. Risk factors for stroke and efficacy of antithrombotic therapy in atrial fibrillation. Analysis of pooled data from five randomized controlled trials. *Arch. Intern. Med.* **1994**, *154*, 1449–1457. [CrossRef]
18. International Stroke Trial Collaborative Group. The International Stroke Trial (IST): A randomised trial of aspirin, subcutaneous heparin, both, or neither among 19435 patients with acute ischaemic stroke. International Stroke Trial Collaborative Group. *Lancet* **1997**, *349*, 1569–1581. [CrossRef]
19. Hart, R.G.; Pearce, L.; Aguilar, M.I. Meta-analysis: Antithrombotic Therapy to Prevent Stroke in Patients Who Have Nonvalvular Atrial Fibrillation. *Ann. Intern. Med.* **2007**, *146*, 857–867. [CrossRef]
20. Mohr, J.; Thompson, J.; Lazar, R.; Levin, B.; Sacco, R.; Furie, K.; Kistler, J.; Albers, G.; Pettigrew, L.; Adams, H.; et al. A Comparison of Warfarin and Aspirin for the Prevention of Recurrent Ischemic Stroke. *N. Engl. J. Med.* **2001**, *345*, 1444–1451. [CrossRef]
21. Giugliano, R.P.; Ruff, C.T.; Braunwald, E.; Murphy, S.A.; Wiviott, S.D.; Halperin, J.L.; Waldo, A.L.; Ezekowitz, M.D.; Weitz, J.I.; Špinar, J.; et al. Edoxaban versus Warfarin in Patients with Atrial Fibrillation. *N. Engl. J. Med.* **2013**, *369*, 2093–2104. [CrossRef]
22. Patel, M.R.; Mahaffey, K.W.; Garg, J.; Pan, G.; Singer, D.E.; Hacke, W.; Breithardt, G.; Halperin, J.L.; Hankey, G.J.; Piccini, J.P.; et al. Rivaroxaban versus Warfarin in Nonvalvular Atrial Fibrillation. *N. Engl. J. Med.* **2011**, *365*, 883–891. [CrossRef] [PubMed]
23. Connolly, S.J.; Ezekowitz, M.D.; Yusuf, S.; Eikelboom, J.; Oldgren, J.; Parekh, A.; Pogue, J.; Reilly, P.A.; Themeles, E.; Varrone, J.; et al. Dabigatran versus Warfarin in Patients with Atrial Fibrillation. *N. Engl. J. Med.* **2009**, *361*, 1139–1151. [CrossRef] [PubMed]
24. Stanifer, J.W.; Pokorney, S.D.; Chertow, G.M.; Hohnloser, S.H.; Wojdyla, D.M.; Garonzik, S.; Byon, W.; Hijazi, Z.; Lopes, R.D.; Alexander, J.H.; et al. Apixaban versus Warfarin in Patients with Atrial Fibrillation and Advanced Chronic Kidney Disease. *Circulation* **2020**, *141*, 1384–1392. [CrossRef] [PubMed]
25. Ruff, C.T.; Giugliano, R.P.; Braunwald, E.; Hoffman, E.B.; Deenadayalu, N.; Ezekowitz, M.D.; Camm, A.J.; Weitz, J.I.; Lewis, B.S.; Parkhomenko, A.; et al. Comparison of the efficacy and safety of new oral anticoagulants with warfarin in patients with atrial fibrillation: A meta-analysis of randomised trials. *Lancet* **2014**, *383*, 955–962. [CrossRef]
26. Eikelboom, J.W.; Connolly, S.J.; Bosch, J.; Dagenais, G.R.; Hart, R.G.; Shestakovska, O.; Diaz, R.; Alings, M.; Lonn, E.M.; Anand, S.S.; et al. Rivaroxaban with or without Aspirin in Stable Cardiovascular Disease. *N. Engl. J. Med.* **2017**, *377*, 1319–1330. [CrossRef]
27. Sharma, M.; Hart, R.G.; Connolly, S.J.; Bosch, J.; Shestakovska, O.; Ng, K.K.H.; Catanese, L.; Keltai, K.; Aboyans, V.; Alings, M.; et al. Stroke Outcomes in the COMPASS Trial. *Circulation* **2019**, *139*, 1134–1145. [CrossRef]
28. Piccini, J.P.; Caso, V.; Connolly, S.J.; Fox, K.A.A.; Oldgren, J.; Jones, W.S.; Gorog, D.A.; Durdil, V.; Viethen, T.; Neumann, C.; et al. Safety of the oral factor XIa inhibitor asundexian compared with apixaban in patients with atrial fibrillation (PACIFIC-AF): A multicentre, randomised, double-blind, double-dummy, dose-finding phase 2 study. *Lancet* **2022**, *399*, 1383–1390. [CrossRef]
29. Chao, W.H. Thrombosis of the left internal carotid artery. *Arch. Surg.* **1938**, *37*, 100–111. [CrossRef]

30. Carrea, R.; Molins, M.; Murphy, G. Surgery of spontaneous thrombosis of the internal carotid in the neck; carotido-carotid anastomosis; case report and analysis of the literature on surgical cases. *Medicina* **1955**, *15*, 20–29.
31. DeBakey, M.E. Successful Carotid Endarterectomy For Cerebrovascular Insufficiency. *JAMA* **1975**, *233*, 1083. [CrossRef] [PubMed]
32. Fields, W.S.; Maslenikov, V.; Meyer, J.S.; Hass, W.K.; Remington, R.D.; Macdonald, M. Joint study of extracranial arterial occlusion. V. Progress report of prognosis following surgery or nonsurgical treatment for transient cerebral ischemic attacks and cervical carotid artery lesions. *JAMA* **1970**, *211*, 1993–2003. [CrossRef] [PubMed]
33. North American Symptomatic Carotid Endarterectomy Trial Collaborators. Beneficial Effect of Carotid Endarterectomy in Symptomatic Patients with High-Grade Carotid Stenosis. *N. Engl. J. Med.* **1991**, *325*, 445–453. [CrossRef] [PubMed]
34. European Carotid Surgery Trialists' Collaborative Group. MRC European Carotid Surgery Trial: Interim results for symptomatic patients with severe (70–99%) or with mild (0–29%) carotid stenosis. *Lancet* **1991**, *337*, 1235–1243. [CrossRef]
35. Paciaroni, M.; Bogousslavsky, J. Chapter 1 The history of stroke and cerebrovascular disease. *Handb. Clin. Neurol.* **2008**, *92*, 3–28. [CrossRef]
36. Esunge, P.M. From Blood Pressure to Hypertension: The History of Research. *J. R. Soc. Med.* **1991**, *84*, 621–621. [CrossRef]
37. Pound, P.; Bury, M.; Ebrahim, S. From apoplexy to stroke. *Age Ageing* **1997**, *26*, 331–337. [CrossRef]
38. Taguchi, J.; Freis, E.D. Partial Reduction of Blood Pressure and Prevention of Complications in Hypertension. *N. Engl. J. Med.* **1974**, *291*, 329–331. [CrossRef]
39. Collins, R.; Peto, R.; MacMahon, S.; Godwin, J.; Qizilbash, N.; Hebert, P.; Eberlein, K.; Taylor, J.; Hennekens, C.; Fiebach, N. Blood pressure, stroke, and coronary heart disease: Part 2, short-term reductions in blood pressure: Overview of randomised drug trials in their epidemiological context. *Lancet* **1990**, *335*, 827–838. [CrossRef]
40. SHEP Cooperative Research Group. Prevention of stroke by antihypertensive drug treatment in older persons with isolated systolic hypertension. Final results of the Systolic Hypertension in the Elderly Program (SHEP). *JAMA* **1991**, *265*, 3255–3264. [CrossRef]
41. Staessen, J.A.; Fagard, R.; Thijs, L.; Celis, H.; Arabidze, G.G.; Birkenhäger, W.H.; Bulpitt, C.J.; de Leeuw, P.W.; Dollery, C.T.; Fletcher, A.E.; et al. Randomised double-blind comparison of placebo and active treatment for older patients with isolated systolic hypertension. *Lancet* **1997**, *350*, 757–764. [CrossRef] [PubMed]
42. Yusuf, S.; Sleight, P.; Pogue, J.F.; Bosch, J.; Davies, R.; Dagenais, G. Effects of an angiotensin-converting-enzyme inhibitor, ramipril, on cardiovascular events in high-risk patients. *N. Engl. J. Med.* **2000**, *342*, 145–153. [PubMed]
43. Group, P.C. Randomised trial of a perindopril-based blood-pressure-lowering regimen among 6,105 individuals with previous stroke or transient ischaemic attack. *Lancet* **2001**, *358*, 1033–1041.
44. World Health Organization; International Society of Hypertension Writing Group. 2003 World Health Organization (WHO)/International Society of Hypertension (ISH) statement on management of hypertension. *J. Hypertens.* **2003**, *21*, 1983–1992. [CrossRef] [PubMed]

45. Chobanian, A.V.; Bakris, G.L.; Black, H.R.; Cushman, W.C.; Green, L.A.; Izzo, J.L., Jr.; Jones, D.W.; Materson, B.J.; Oparil, S.; Wright, J.T., Jr.; et al. Seventh Report of the Joint National Committee on Prevention, Detection, Evaluation, and Treatment of High Blood Pressure. *Hypertension* **2003**, *42*, 1206–1252. [CrossRef]
46. European Society of Hypertension-European Society of Cardiology Guidelines Committee. 2003 European Society of Hypertension-European Society of Cardiology guidelines for the management of arterial hypertension. *J. Hypertens.* **2003**, *21*, 1011–1053. [CrossRef]
47. Chalmers, J.; MacMahon, S. PROGRESS in Blood Pressure Control for the Prevention of Secondary Stroke. *Cerebrovasc. Dis.* **2021**, *50*, 617–621. [CrossRef]
48. Bushnell, C.; McCullough, L.D.; Awad, I.A.; Chireau, M.V.; Fedder, W.N.; Furie, K.L.; Howard, V.J.; Lichtman, J.H.; Lisabeth, L.D.; Piña, I.L.; et al. Guidelines for the prevention of stroke in women: A statement for healthcare professionals from the American Heart Association/American Stroke Association. *Stroke* **2014**, *45*, 1545–1588. [CrossRef]
49. Wann, S.; Thomas, G.S. What can ancient mummies teach us about atherosclerosis? *Trends Cardiovasc. Med.* **2014**, *24*, 279–284. [CrossRef]
50. Olson, R.E. Discovery of the Lipoproteins, Their Role in Fat Transport and Their Significance as Risk Factors. *J. Nutr.* **1998**, *128* (Suppl. 2), S439–S443. [CrossRef]
51. Endo, A. A historical perspective on the discovery of statins. *Proc. Jpn. Acad. Ser. B Phys. Biol. Sci.* **2010**, *86*, 484–493. [CrossRef]
52. Siri-Tarino, P.W.; Krauss, R.M. The early years of lipoprotein research: From discovery to clinical application. *J. Lipid Res.* **2016**, *57*, 1771–1777. [CrossRef]
53. Kuijpers, P.M.J.C. History in Medicine: The Story of Cholesterol, Lipids and Cardiology. 2021. Available online: https://www.escardio.org/Journals/E-Journal-of-Cardiology-Practice/Volume-19/history-in-medicine-the-story-of-cholesterol-lipids-and-cardiology (accessed on 4 April 2022).
54. The Stroke Prevention by Aggressive Reduction in Cholesterol Levels (SPARCL) Investigators. High-dose atorvastatin after stroke or transient ischemic attack. *N. Engl. J. Med.* **2006**, *355*, 549–559. [CrossRef]
55. Amarenco, P.; Kim, J.S.; Labreuche, J.; Charles, H.; Abtan, J.; Béjot, Y.; Cabrejo, L.; Cha, J.-K.; Ducrocq, G.; Giroud, M.; et al. A Comparison of Two LDL Cholesterol Targets after Ischemic Stroke. *N. Engl. J. Med.* **2020**, *382*, 9–19. [CrossRef]
56. Azarpazhooh, M.R.; Bogiatzi, C.; Spence, J.D. Stroke Prevention: Little-Known and Neglected Aspects. *Cerebrovasc. Dis.* **2021**, *50*, 622–635. [CrossRef]
57. Mach, F.; Baigent, C.; Catapano, A.L.; Koskinas, K.C.; Casula, M.; Badimon, L.; Chapman, M.J.; De Backer, G.G.; Delgado, V.; Ference, B.A.; et al. 2019 ESC/EAS Guidelines for the management of dyslipidaemias: Lipid modification to reduce cardiovascular risk. *Eur. Heart J.* **2020**, *41*, 111–188. [CrossRef]
58. Kim, E.J.; Wierzbicki, A.S. The history of proprotein convertase subtilisin kexin-9 inhibitors and their role in the treatment of cardiovascular disease. *Ther. Adv. Chronic Dis.* **2020**, *11*, 2040622320924569. [CrossRef] [PubMed]

59. Bonaca, M.P.; Nault, P.; Giugliano, R.P.; Keech, A.C.; Pineda, A.L.; Kanevsky, E.; Kuder, J.; Murphy, S.A.; Jukema, J.W.; Lewis, B.S.; et al. Low-Density Lipoprotein Cholesterol Lowering with Evolocumab and Outcomes in Patients with Peripheral Artery Disease: Insights From the FOURIER Trial (Further Cardiovascular Outcomes Research with PCSK9 Inhibition in Subjects with Elevated Risk). *Circulation* **2018**, *137*, 338–350. [CrossRef] [PubMed]
60. Farnier, M.; Jones, P.; Severance, R.; Averna, M.; Steinhagen-Thiessen, E.; Colhoun, H.M.; Du, Y.; Hanotin, C.; Donahue, S. Efficacy and safety of adding alirocumab to rosuvastatin versus adding ezetimibe or doubling the rosuvastatin dose in high cardiovascular-risk patients: The ODYSSEY OPTIONS II randomized trial. *Atherosclerosis* **2016**, *244*, 138–146. [CrossRef]
61. Lakhtakia, R. The history of diabetes mellitus. *Sultan Qaboos Univ. Med. J.* **2013**, *13*, 368–370. [CrossRef] [PubMed]
62. Allan, F.N. Diabetes before and after insulin. *Med. Hist.* **1972**, *16*, 266–273. [CrossRef] [PubMed]
63. Diabetes Control and Complications Trial Research Group. The effect of intensive treatment of diabetes on the development and progression of long-term complications in insulin-dependent diabetes mellitus. *N. Engl. J. Med.* **1993**, *329*, 977–986. [CrossRef] [PubMed]
64. Harold, J.G. Harold on History: An Historical Perspective on Diabetes and Cardiovascular Disease. 2017. Available online: https://www.acc.org/latest-in-cardiology/articles/2017/08/16/10/42/harold-on-history-an-historical-perspective-on-diabetes-and-cardiovascular-disease (accessed on 25 January 2022.).
65. Gerstein, H.C.; Hart, R.; Colhoun, H.M.; Diaz, R.; Lakshmanan, M.; Botros, F.T.; Probstfield, J.; Riddle, M.C.; Rydén, L.; Atisso, C.M.; et al. The effect of dulaglutide on stroke: An exploratory analysis of the REWIND trial. *Lancet Diabetes Endocrinol.* **2020**, *8*, 106–114. [CrossRef] [PubMed]
66. Malhotra, K.; Katsanos, A.H.; Lambadiari, V.; Goyal, N.; Palaiodimou, L.; Kosmidou, M.; Krogias, C.; Alexandrov, A.V.; Tsivgoulis, G. GLP-1 receptor agonists in diabetes for stroke prevention: A systematic review and meta-analysis. *J. Neurol.* **2020**, *267*, 2117–2122. [CrossRef]
67. Yaghi, S.; Furie, K.L.; Viscoli, C.M.; Kamel, H.; Gorman, M.; Dearborn, J.; Young, L.H.; Inzucchi, S.E.; Lovejoy, A.M.; Kasner, S.E.; et al. Pioglitazone Prevents Stroke in Patients with a Recent Transient Ischemic Attack or Ischemic Stroke: A Planned Secondary Analysis of the IRIS Trial (Insulin Resistance Intervention After Stroke). *Circulation* **2018**, *137*, 455–463. [CrossRef]
68. GBD 2019 Stroke Collaborators. Global, regional, and national burden of stroke and its risk factors, 1990–2019: A systematic analysis for the Global Burden of Disease Study 2019. *Lancet Neurol.* **2021**, *20*, 795–820. [CrossRef]

© 2023 by the authors. Licensee MDPI, Basel, Switzerland. This article is an open access article distributed under the terms and conditions of the Creative Commons Attribution (CC BY) license (http://creativecommons.org/licenses/by/4.0/).

History of Stroke Imaging

Michael G. Hennerici and Stephen Meairs

Abstract: This chapter summarizes the history of cerebrovascular brain imaging from its early roots (clinical anatomy) in the 17th century to the first successful technological steps and the application of various brain and vessel imaging procedures in the last two centuries. Today, cerebrovascular ultrasound, cranial computed tomography and magnetic resonance brain imaging all contribute to our current diagnostic management for the best early stroke treatment in the acute phase with high-technology expertise.

1. Early Progress in Understanding Stroke—The Need for Brain Imaging

Although some signs and symptoms of permanent stroke were already known in ancient Egyptian, Greek and Roman times, many were sources of misinterpretation among a wide variety of established knowledge. Hippocrates created the term apoplexy—still misused today even in medical books and scientific writing—for a sudden condition of a disease, later termed as stroke, referring to a sudden or chronic interrupted blood supply to specific areas of the brain. The treatment and prevention of stroke were extremely limited, as written in Galen's *Opera Omina*, published in Venice in 1556: *"It is impossible to cure a severe attack of apoplexy and difficult to cure a mild one"*.

Progress in understanding stroke was made in the 17th century. Thomas Willis (1621–1675), an English physician who was born near and practiced in Oxford as a local physician, was known as one of the first pioneers in our present knowledge of the anatomy of the brain and associated brain diseases. Apart from his achievement as the first to describe cerebral circulation, and having the circle of Willis named after his identification, he also described the twelve brain nerves and coined the term *neurology*. Willis discussed many signs and symptoms of behavioral and functional neurological problems which are still known and identified today. In 1658, Johann Jakob Wepfer (1620–1695) (Figure 1), a physician in Schaffhausen, Switzerland, identified the main causes of stroke as ischemia and hemorrhage, based on post-mortem examinations of people who died of the condition.

In spite of the increasing knowledge regarding the pathophysiology of stroke, there remained no means of clinical verification of this condition, especially with respect to etiology. An instrument to assess the cerebral vasculature or to image brain ischemia and hemorrhage was lacking, and this deficit continued for centuries!

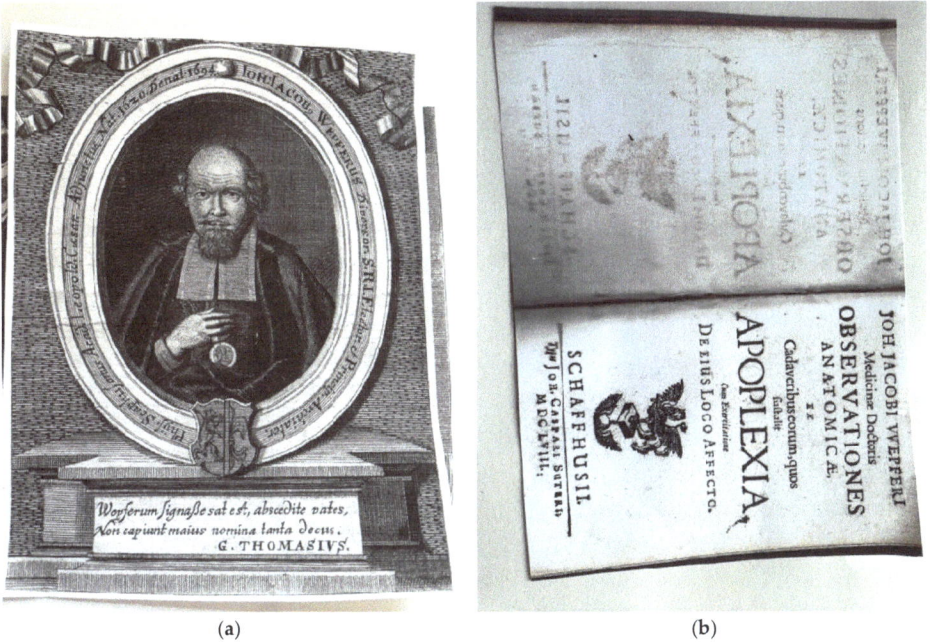

Figure 1. (a) Johann Jakob Wepfer (1620–1695). (b) *Observationes anatomicae, ex cadaveribus eorum, quos sustulit apoplexia.* Source: private library of Michael Hennerici.

2. Computed Tomography

The invention and development of computed tomography (CT) is a fascinating story in the history of medicine. It includes one of the 20th century's most important music recording companies and a Nobel laureate in medicine and physiology who never attended medical school or earned a PhD. In the 1960s, Godfrey Hounsfield was employed as an electrical engineer by Electric and Music Industries (EMI), the company that would become better known for recording and selling the Beatles' albums. Hounsfield proposed to his company that he develop a machine that would be capable of imaging the human brain. Although EMI had no experience in manufacturing medical equipment, the company agreed to support Hounsfield's idea to realize a totally new approach to medical imaging with X-rays. The first CT scanner, designed specifically for the examination of the brain, was installed at the Atkinson Morley Hospital in Wimbledon, England. On 1 October 1971, the first CT scan of a human patient revealed a clinically suspected brain tumor. Indeed, Hounsfield's innovation transformed medicine. He shared the Nobel Prize for Physiology or Medicine in 1979 and was knighted by Queen Elizabeth II in 1981.

EMI distributed a number of machines to the United States, the first to the Mayo Clinic. By 1973, Ambrose had already reported on the usefulness of the EMI scanner for the depiction of brain infarction, hemorrhage and edema [1], thus paving the way for new developments in the field of clinical stroke research. Using an EM1 Mark I modified 160 x 160 matrix scanner, neurologists at Harvard reported the visualization of large confluent petechial hemorrhages and/or hemorrhage within infarcts, noting that sequential CT changes in infarcts correlated well with established pathologic changes [2].

The first EMI scanner was quite slow (5 minutes per image acquisition) and had a low image resolution. It required the use of a water-filled tank with a pre-shaped rubber "head-cap" at the front, which enclosed the patient's head. This feature was prohibitive for further developments, especially with respect to whole body scanning. The prototype Automatic Computerized Transverse Axial scanner (ACTA), designed by Robert Ledley at Georgetown University, was acquired by the Pfizer drug company, along with the rights to manufacture it. ACTA produced images in a 256 × 256 matrix, which only took about 20 seconds to acquire. This whole-body scanner was widely distributed over the next few years.

A major milestone in technological advances of CT was the spiral-CT, invented by Will Kalendar in Germany. The first CT scanner to implement this technique was the Siemens Somatom Plus. Within a short time, all other manufacturers had implemented this technology in their CT machines. Major benefits included a reduced scanning time, multi-slice capability, a reduction in movement artifacts, and isotrope voxels. In 2005, Siemens introduced a dual-source CT which offered a further significant reduction in scan time.

The long-awaited ability to image stroke had finally become a reality. In the following years, the enormous progress made in CT technology allowed physicians to quickly and reliably discern

(a) Whether signs and symptoms were related to ischemic or hemorrhagic stroke;
(b) Whether an ischemic stroke was arterial or embolic;
(c) Which regions of the brain were involved;
(d) Whether structures of the brain were already dead, at risk or not yet involved.

CT provided the first diagnostic platform for making clinical decisions on whether to treat stroke patients with thrombolytic drugs. While CT has a relatively low sensitivity for the detection of brain ischemia, it depicts irreversible tissue damage with high specificity. CT reliably detects brain hemorrhage, a contraindication for thrombolysis. In addition, the extent of CT hypoattenuation is an important positive predictor of thrombolysis-induced brain hemorrhage, the most feared complication of thrombolysis.

Research by the Belgian molecular biologist Desire Collen supported the idea of ischemic stroke treatment in his search for a way to dissolve blood clots. He developed a substance best known today as alteplase recombinant tissue plasminogen activator (rt-PA), which can dismantle the underlying framework of a clot/thrombus and break it down. Clinical trials with rt-PA were undertaken in the early 1980s for coronary and deep vein thrombolysis. Only possible through the CT imaging of suspected acute brain infarction, the first results from multicenter studies of intravenous rt-PA therapy in stroke were reported in 1990 [3]. Today, treatment with rt-PA is standardized not only within 4.5 hours after stroke onset, as initially approved, but also for wake-up stroke with an unknown time of onset during sleep in MRI-guided stroke evaluation [4].

The addition of *CT perfusion imaging* and *CT angiography* allowed for a positive diagnosis of ischemic stroke versus mimics and for the identification of a large vessel occlusion target for endovascular thrombectomy. CT perfusion imaging can also provide imaging evidence of salvageable brain tissue, thus facilitating decision making in late recanalization strategies.

In 2010, Klaus Fassender's team at the University Hospital of the Saarland in Germany reported on the first mobile stroke unit using a *mobile CT scanner* from Philips [5]. This unit consisted of an ambulance equipped with the CT scanner, a point-of-care laboratory system for complete stroke laboratory work-up, and telemedicine capabilities for contact with hospital experts. The mobile stroke unit achieved the delivery of etiology-specific and guideline-adherent stroke treatment at the site of the emergency, well before arrival at the hospital. In a departure from current practice, stroke patients could be differentially treated according to their ischemic or hemorrhagic etiology even in the pre-hospital phase of stroke management. The immediate diagnosis of cerebral ischemia and the exclusion of thrombolysis contraindications enabled prehospital rt-PA thrombolysis.

3. Magnetic Resonance Imaging

In the 1990s, magnetic resonance imaging (MRI) emerged as a clinically useful diagnostic modality for stroke and other neurologic disorders [6,7]. In the detection of ischemic stroke lesions, MRI was more sensitive than CT, particularly for small infarcts and in sites such as the cerebellum and brainstem and deep white matter [8].Conventional MRI techniques such as *T1-weighted imaging* and *fluid-attenuated inversion recovery imaging* reliably detected ischemic parenchymal changes beyond the first 12 to 24 hours after onset. These methods were combined with *MR angiography* to noninvasively assess the intracranial and extracranial vasculature. However, MRI could not yet adequately assess the extent and severity of ischemic changes within the critical first 3 to 6 hours, the period of greatest therapeutic opportunity.

The revolutionary development of *diffusion-weighted imaging* (DWI) sequences allowed the imaging of cerebral ischemic events within the first 6 hours from onset [9], thus offering immense potential clinical utility in the early detection and investigation of patients with stroke. Further technical developments such as echoplanar imaging made the diffusion and perfusion of MRI feasible in routine clinical practice. A further milestone was the detection of hyperacute intraparenchymal hemorrhagic stroke using *susceptibility-weighted MRI*, which proved to be comparable to CT [10]. Thus, in combination with MR angiography, a multimodal MRI exam allowed for the detection of the site, age, extent, mechanism and tissue viability of acute stroke lesions in a single imaging study. This revolution in stroke imaging allowed therapeutic and clinical decisions to be based on the physiologic state of cerebral tissue. Moreover, this new methodology proved capable as a patient selection tool for experimental and interventional therapies, and as a biomarker of therapeutic response in clinical trials.

4. Cerebrovascular Ultrasound

Ultrasound has played an important role in the evaluation of both early and advanced atherosclerotic disease, in the identification of stroke etiology and in the monitoring of stroke patients. From a historical perspective, its relative importance to other stroke imaging modalities, particularly those of CT and MRI, has somewhat declined. This is due predominantly to an emphasis upon new treatment strategies implementing acute endovascular thrombectomy, which is guided by the simultaneous use of brain and vascular imaging techniques. Although European centers continue to stress the need for transcranial Doppler and carotid duplex sonography in the accreditation of stroke units, current American stroke guidelines lack defining indications for these ultrasound techniques. Nevertheless, there remains an additional clinical contribution of neurovascular ultrasound in the post-acute care management of patients with acute ischemic stroke and in preventive and follow-up studies.

Continuous wave (CW) Doppler was the earliest ultrasound technique used to assess carotid stenosis, a common cause of stroke. The Doppler effect is named after Christian Doppler, who in 1842 described the change in frequency of light emitted by moving objects. This effect is familiar to anyone who has stood in one place and listened to a source of sound passing by. The sound rises in pitch as the source approaches the listener and then equally drops off as the source moves away after passing. In clinical applications, this effect is known as the Doppler frequency shift, which is the difference between emitted and received ultrasonography frequency and is proportional to the velocity of moving blood cells.

In 1956, Shigeo Satomura (1919–1960), a physicist at Osaka University, made one of the greatest contributions to the field of diagnostic ultrasound when he discovered that the Doppler principle could be applied to ultrasonic energy [11]. Satomura applied the Doppler effect to develop the 'Ultrasonic Blood Rheograph', which was then manufactured as the first commercial ultrasonic Doppler flowmeter by the Nippon Electric Company in 1959. In collaboration with the neurologist Ziro Kaneko (1915–1997), Satomura distinguished arterial flow into high- and low-resistance vasculatures, and then showed in 1962 that the Doppler signal actually arose from the backscattered energy from the moving blood cells [12].

The important discovery by Satomura led to the development of continuous wave (CW) Doppler systems, which use two transducers, one of which emits while the other receives ultrasound continuously. CW Doppler of the ophthalmic artery was one of the earliest methods used as an indirect test for the detection of significant carotid artery stenosis [13]. This periorbital technique provided information about the existence of collateral pathways. In the presence of severe stenosis or the occlusion of the internal carotid artery (ICA), retrograde blood supply from the external carotid artery via the ophthalmic anastomosis was easily detected using CW Doppler. However, with sufficient collateralization from the contralateral carotid artery or the vertebrobasilar systems, the orthograde perfusion of the ophthalmic artery could occur. Thus, this indirect test could not detect hemodynamically significant ipsilateral carotid obstruction in up to 20% of patients.

CW Doppler ultrasound for the direct detection of ICA stenosis was reported in 1968 [14]. Although this method detected a broad range of changes in flow velocity associated with carotid stenosis, it provided only limited information on the actual origin of the ultrasound reflecting source. Later, *pulsed-wave (PW) Doppler* systems, in which ultrasound is both emitted from and received by a single piezoelectric crystal in the transducer, were able to provide a depth estimate of the site being insonated [12].

Duplex ultrasonography was a significant imaging milestone in the history of stroke imaging. It combined integrated PW Doppler spectrum analysis and *B-mode scanning*, which displays the morphologic features of normal and diseased vessels. The B-mode image served as a guide for the placement of the PW Doppler sample volume. The Doppler spectrum analysis provided criteria for evaluation of hemodynamics and for the categorization of ICA stenoses.

Although both CW and PW Doppler techniques were simple, inexpensive screening procedures for the detection of stenoses and occlusions in the extracranial arteries, they were largely replaced by *color Doppler flow imaging (CDFI)*, which preserved the advantages of duplex ultrasonography and superimposed color-coded blood flow patterns onto the gray-scale B-mode image. With the use of a defined color scale, the direction and the average mean velocity of moving blood cells within the sample volume at a given point in time were encoded, thus allowing the real-time visualization of hemodynamics. CDFI provided an excellent evaluation of extracranial arteries and was later adapted in transcranial applications. Special transducers were developed to assess the distal extracranial lesions of the ICA, such as carotid dissections, fibromuscular dysplasia, and atypically located atherosclerosis [12,15].

Pioneer studies by Hennerici et al. in 1981 provided ultrasound documentation of the incidence of asymptomatic carotid stenosis [16]. Further work resulted in the first report of the natural history of carotid stenosis [17]. Numerous studies reported on the use of ultrasound to identify symptomatic or vulnerable carotid artery plaques. Parameters for classification included echogenicity, surface structure, and ulcerations [12].

An important milestone in stroke prevention was the demonstration that the first morphological abnormalities of arterial walls can be visualized by B-mode ultrasonography. In 1986, Pignoli and coworkers characterized a "double-line" pattern of the normal carotid artery wall with B-mode ultrasonography [18]. They described the first echogenic line on the far wall to represent the lumen–intima interface and the second line to correspond to the media–adventitia interface.

Significantly, they demonstrated that the distance between these two echogenic lines correlated highly with measurements of intima-media thickness (IMT) in tissue specimens from common carotid arteries. Pignoli's initial report on the measurement of IMT with B-mode scanning was later validated in vitro [19] and was shown to enable good intra-observer and inter-observer reproducibility [12,20].

In the following years, technological advances in B-mode ultrasonography led to a high-resolution, noninvasive technique that offered an excellent method for the detection of early stages of atherosclerotic disease. This success was based upon its simple nature, wide availability, and capacity to depict arterial wall structures with better resolution than other imaging techniques (e.g., MRI or CT). Accordingly, many studies consequently used high-resolution ultrasonography to establish associations between common carotid IMT, cardiovascular risk factors, and the prevalence of cardiovascular disease. The importance of common carotid IMT is reflected by its use as a surrogate endpoint [12]. Important guidelines for the standardization of carotid IMT measurements and the classification of early atherosclerotic lesions were offered by the Mannheim carotid intima-media thickness and plaque consensus meetings from 2004 to 2011 [21].

In 1982, Aaslid et al. described noninvasive *transcranial Doppler (TCD)* for depicting flow velocities in the basal cerebral arteries [22]. TCD later evolved into applications for the detection of intracranial stenosis and occlusion (the sensitivity for the detection of MCA occlusion by TCD was about 80% with a high specificity [15]), the evaluation of intracranial collateral circulations, the detection of vasospasm in subarachnoid hemorrhage (SAH), the assessment of cerebral autoregulation, and for the surveillance of intracranial hemodynamics during stroke therapy.

TCD detection of *high intensity transient signals (HITS)* entering the cerebral circulation was first reported in 1986 [23]. This important discovery led to studies showing how this technique could be used to identify microembolic signals in patients who may be at increased risk for stroke. HITS corresponding to both gaseous and solid microembolic materials were reported during angiography, carotid angioplasty, open heart surgery, and carotid endarterectomy, as well as in patients with TIAs or stroke, asymptomatic carotid stenosis, heart valve prosthesis, and intracranial arterial disease [12].

Because *brain perfusion imaging* may detect ischemic lesions earlier than CT and may distinguish the stroke subtype and severity of cerebral ischemia, there was great interest in the use of perfusion imaging to predict recovery, differentiate stroke pathogenesis, and monitor therapy. Advanced contrast-specific ultrasound imaging technologies were developed for the assessment of brain perfusion in stroke patients [12,24].

Most studies of cerebral perfusion with ultrasound imaging applied a high mechanical index (MI) after the injection of microbubbles (MBs) as a contrast agent. The MI is a measure of acoustic output. Since MBs are destroyed in the cerebral microcirculation with high MI imaging, a triggered pulsing sequence was implemented to allow for the replenishment of new MBs in the ultrasound scan plane. Accordingly, most early studies of cerebral perfusion were performed with triggered harmonic gray scale imaging techniques (conventional, power modulation or pulse-inversion) analyzing the bolus kinetics in healthy subjects to determine the best method for the detection of MBs in the cerebral microcirculation [12].

Sophisticated *low-MI real time perfusion* techniques were later introduced, which allowed the detection of MB in the cerebral microcirculation without destruction, as compared to the high MI-imaging. This allowed the application of a high frame rate, which led to a better time resolution of bolus kinetics. Low-MI ultrasound imaging was used to monitor MB replenishment in real time following the application of destruction pulses at high MI [25]. The behavior of the refill kinetics was assessed with an exponential curve fit, which provided parameters for the analysis of cerebral blood flow.

Since individual MBs could be depicted flowing through small vessels in the brain with low MI imaging, it was possible to track these bubbles and map perfusion over time. Dynamic microvascular MB maps provided a demarcation of MCA infarctions and impressive displays of low velocity tissue MB refill following destruction with high mechanical index imaging.

A highly interesting development in the history of ultrasound was the discovery that it might not only be effective for imaging, but also for stroke therapy. Indeed, in vitro experiments and animal studies indicated that ultrasound together with thrombolytic therapy, *sonothrombolysis*, improved the recanalization of occluded intracerebral vessels [26]. Moreover, it was later shown that ultrasound together with microbubbles alone could foster recanalization, thus opening the possibility for a new approach to clot lysis without thrombolytic drugs [12].

CLOTBUST (Combined Lysis of Thrombus in Brain Ischemia Using Transcranial Ultrasound and Systemic tPA) [27] was a multi-center randomized clinical trial of patients with acute ischemic stroke due to MCA occlusion. Target patients received, along with tPA, 2-MHz, pulsed wave transcranial Doppler monitoring for a duration of two hours. A complete reperfusion or dramatic clinical recovery was observed for 49% of the patients in the target group (tPA+US) and for only 30% of the control group. The TRUMBI trial (Transcranial Low-Frequency Ultrasound-Mediated Thrombolysis in Brain Ischemia) was stopped prematurely because of the occurrence of a higher number of intracerebral hemorrhages after tPA treatment combined with transcranial sonication at 300 kHz [28]. Unfortunately, later large-scale studies implementing ultrasound at clinical monitoring frequencies were unable to confirm a positive effect of sonothrombolysis.

Any history of stroke imaging would be incomplete without acknowledging how stroke conferences served to shape and nurture imaging modalities for clinical applications. This was not only true for the fertilization of concerted research activities, but also for developing standards for stroke imaging in diagnosis, follow-up and prevention. Meetings of the American Stroke Association and the European Stroke Conference set the stage for regular scientific exchange among clinicians and researchers interested in the pathophysiology, diagnosis and treatment of cerebrovascular diseases throughout the world. These conferences were instrumental in promoting international dialogue, and served as platforms for the communication of various stroke organizations and, importantly, for the initiation of many international research activities. Key speakers were often well-known imaging experts, and stroke imaging sessions were highlights of these conferences, which led to the rapid communication of state-of-the-art imaging procedures [29].

Funding: This research received no external funding.

Conflicts of Interest: The authors declare no conflict of interest.

References

1. Ambrose, J.A. The usefulness of computerized transverse axial scanning in problems arising from cerebral haemorrhage, infarction or oedema. *Br. J. Radiol.* **1973**, *46*, 736.
2. Davis, K.R.; Ackerman, R.H.; Kistler, J.P.; Mohr, J.P. Computed tomography of cerebral infarction: Hemorrhagic, contrast enhancement, and time of appearance. *Comput. Tomogr.* **1977**, *1*, 71–86. [CrossRef]
3. del Zoppo, G.J. An open, multicenter trial of recombinant tissue plasminogen activator in acute stroke. A progress report. The rt-PA Acute Stroke Study Group. *Stroke* **1990**, *21*, IV174–IV175.
4. Thomalla, G.; Simonsen, C.Z.; Boutitie, F.; Andersen, G.; Berthezene, Y.; Cheng, B.; Cheripelli, B.; Cho, T.H.; Fazekas, F.; Fiehler, J.; et al. MRI-Guided Thrombolysis for Stroke with Unknown Time of Onset. *N. Engl. J. Med.* **2018**, *379*, 611–622. [CrossRef]
5. Walter, S.; Kostpopoulos, P.; Haass, A.; Helwig, S.; Keller, I.; Licina, T.; Schlechtriemen, T.; Roth, C.; Papanagiotou, P.; Zimmer, A.; et al. Bringing the hospital to the patient: First treatment of stroke patients at the emergency site. *PLoS ONE* **2010**, *5*, e13758. [CrossRef]
6. Bydder, G.M.; Steiner, R.E.; Young, I.R.; Hall, A.S.; Thomas, D.J.; Marshall, J.; Pallis, C.A.; Legg, N.J. Clinical NMR imaging of the brain: 140 cases. *AJR Am. J. Roentgenol.* **1982**, *139*, 215–236. [CrossRef]
7. Buonanno, F.S.; Kistler, J.P.; DeWitt, L.D.; Pykett, I.L.; Brady, T.J. Proton (1H) nuclear magnetic resonance (NMR) imaging in stroke syndromes. *Neurol. Clin.* **1983**, *1*, 243–262. [CrossRef]
8. Bogousslavsky, J.; Fox, A.J.; Barnett, H.J.; Hachinski, V.C.; Vinitski, S.; Carey, L.S. Clinico-topographic correlation of small vertebrobasilar infarct using magnetic resonance imaging. *Stroke* **1986**, *17*, 929–938. [CrossRef]
9. Le Bihan, D.; Breton, E.; Lallemand, D.; Grenier, P.; Cabanis, E.; Laval-Jeantet, M. MR imaging of intravoxel incoherent motions: Application to diffusion and perfusion in neurologic disorders. *Radiology* **1986**, *161*, 401–407. [CrossRef]
10. Kidwell, C.S.; Chalela, J.A.; Saver, J.L.; Starkman, S.; Hill, M.D.; Demchuk, A.M.; Butman, J.A.; Patronas, N.; Alger, J.R.; Latour, L.L.; et al. Comparison of MRI and CT for detection of acute intracerebral hemorrhage. *JAMA* **2004**, *292*, 1823–1830. [CrossRef]
11. White, D.N. Neurosonology pioneers. *Ultrasound Med. Biol.* **1988**, *14*, 541–561. [CrossRef] [PubMed]

12. Meairs, S.; Hennerici, M.; Mohr, J.P. Ultrasonography. In *Stroke*, 5th ed.; Mohr, J.P., Wolf, P.A., Moskowitz, M.A., Mayberg, M., Grotta, J.C., Eds.; WB Saunders: Philadelphia, PA, USA, 2011; pp. 831–869.
13. Maroon, J.C.; Pieroni, D.W.; Campbell, R.L. Ophthalmosonometry. An ultrasonic method for assessing carotid blood flow. *J. Neurosurg.* **1969**, *30*, 238–246. [CrossRef]
14. Brinker, R.A.; Landiss, D.J.; Croley, T.F. Detection of carotid artery bifurcation stenosis by Doppler ultrasound. Preliminary report. *J. Neurosurg.* **1968**, *29*, 143–148. [CrossRef] [PubMed]
15. Hennerici, M.; Neuerburg-Heusler, D. *Vascular Diagnosis with Ultrasound*; Thieme Publ.: Stuttgart, Germany; New York, NY, USA, 1998.
16. Hennerici, M.; Aulich, A.; Sandmann, W.; Freund, H.J. Incidence of asymptomatic extracranial arterial disease. *Stroke* **1981**, *12*, 750–758. [CrossRef]
17. Hennerici, M.; Rautenberg, W.; Mohr, S. Stroke risk from symptomless extracranial arterial disease. *Lancet* **1982**, *2*, 1180–1183. [CrossRef] [PubMed]
18. Pignoli, P.; Tremoli, E.; Poli, A.; Oreste, P.; Paoletti, R. Intimal plus medial thickness of the arterial wall: A direct measurement with ultrasound imaging. *Circulation* **1986**, *74*, 1399–1406. [CrossRef]
19. Wong, M.; Edelstein, J.; Wollman, J.; Bond, M.G. Ultrasonic-pathological comparison of the human arterial wall. Verification of intima-media thickness. *Arterioscler. Thromb.* **1993**, *13*, 482–486. [CrossRef]
20. Riley, W.A.; Barnes, R.W.; Applegate, W.B.; Dempsey, R.; Hartwell, T.; Davis, V.G.; Bond, M.G.; Furberg, C.D. Reproducibility of noninvasive ultrasonic measurement of carotid atherosclerosis. The Asymptomatic Carotid Artery Plaque Study. *Stroke* **1992**, *23*, 1062–1068. [CrossRef]
21. Touboul, P.J.; Hennerici, M.G.; Meairs, S.; Adams, H.; Amarenco, P.; Bornstein, N.; Csiba, L.; Desvarieux, M.; Ebrahim, S.; Hernandez Hernandez, R.; et al. Mannheim carotid intima-media thickness and plaque consensus (2004–2006–2011). An update on behalf of the advisory board of the 3rd, 4th and 5th watching the risk symposia, at the 13th, 15th and 20th European Stroke Conferences, Mannheim, Germany, 2004, Brussels, Belgium, 2006, and Hamburg, Germany, 2011. *Cerebrovasc. Dis.* **2012**, *34*, 290–296. [CrossRef]
22. Aaslid, R.; Markwalder, T.M.; Nornes, H. Noninvasive transcranial Doppler ultrasound recording of flow velocity in basal cerebral arteries. *J. Neurosurg.* **1982**, *57*, 769–774. [CrossRef]
23. Padayachee, T.S.; Gosling, R.G.; Bishop, C.C.; Burnand, K.; Browse, N.L. Monitoring middle cerebral artery blood velocity during carotid endarterectomy. *Br. J. Surg.* **1986**, *73*, 98–100. [CrossRef] [PubMed]
24. Seidel, G.; Meairs, S. Ultrasound contrast agents in ischemic stroke. *Cerebrovasc. Dis.* **2009**, *27* (Suppl. 2), 25–39. [CrossRef] [PubMed]
25. Kern, R.; Diels, A.; Pettenpohl, J.; Kablau, M.; Brade, J.; Hennerici, M.G.; Meairs, S. Real-time ultrasound brain perfusion imaging with analysis of microbubble replenishment in acute MCA stroke. *J. Cereb. Blood Flow. Metab.* **2011**, *31*, 1716–1724. [CrossRef]
26. Meairs, S.; Alonso, A.; Hennerici, M.G. Progress in sonothrombolysis for the treatment of stroke. *Stroke* **2012**, *43*, 1706–1710. [CrossRef]

27. Alexandrov, A.V.; Molina, C.A.; Grotta, J.C.; Garami, Z.; Ford, S.R.; Alvarez-Sabin, J.; Montaner, J.; Saqqur, M.; Demchuk, A.M.; Moye, L.A.; et al. Ultrasound-enhanced systemic thrombolysis for acute ischemic stroke. *N. Engl. J. Med.* **2004**, *351*, 2170–2178. [CrossRef] [PubMed]
28. Daffertshofer, M.; Gass, A.; Ringleb, P.; Sitzer, M.; Sliwka, U.; Els, T.; Sedlaczek, O.; Koroshetz, W.J.; Hennerici, M.G. Transcranial low-frequency ultrasound-mediated thrombolysis in brain ischemia: Increased risk of hemorrhage with combined ultrasound and tissue plasminogen activator: Results of a phase II clinical trial. *Stroke* **2005**, *36*, 1441–1446. [CrossRef]
29. Mattle, H.P. The Johann Jacob Wepfer Award 2012 of the European Stroke Conference to Professor Louis R. Caplan. *Cerebrovasc. Dis.* **2012**, *34*, 18–19. [CrossRef]

© 2023 by the authors. Licensee MDPI, Basel, Switzerland. This article is an open access article distributed under the terms and conditions of the Creative Commons Attribution (CC BY) license (http://creativecommons.org/licenses/by/4.0/).

Stroke Units, Stroke Registries, and Acute Management (R)evolutions

Carmen Calvello, Lucia Gentili and Roberta Rinaldi

Abstract: Over the past 30 years, stroke units have become the gold standard for inpatient stroke care. Nowadays, all patients hospitalized for stroke should be assessed by trained staff. Improved outcomes have been reported in patients treated in stroke units; therefore, international guidelines were redacted and now highlight that every kind of patient should be treated in stroke units because no subtype, no severity of stroke, and no age group modify the outcomes. These improved outcomes have been assigned to the work of a multidisciplinary team that could better manage early complications. Stroke registers have become a useful tool in clinical practice, facilitating the collection of epidemiological data on stroke and contributing to progressive improvements in the quality of care. There are many ongoing challenges, but the most important contemporary challenge is how to manage stroke unit care in low-income countries.

1. Introduction

Over the past 30 years there has been a revolution in stroke management. The origin of the stroke unit, as a structure capable of welcoming and satisfying the needs of the stroke patient, and the emergence of new professional figures who collaborate in teams have allowed the identification and development of new therapeutic approaches. If once the stroke was interpreted as a "consequence" of progressive cerebral aging, today it represents a neurological disease with some of the greatest therapeutic possibilities able to modify patient outcomes.

2. Stroke Unit Care

2.1. Recent Revolution over the Last 30 Years

During the last few decades of the 20th century, there was a progressive development in the treatment of patients with acute stroke [1].

Stroke was an inevitable event until the mid-1990s; it was believed that medical interventions were little effective, and the absence of dedicated medical specialists determined different management approaches for the disease all over the world.

The development of new vascular imaging techniques, such as computed tomography (CT), magnetic resonance imaging (MRI) and ultrasound (US), highlighted that the diagnosis and treatment of stroke are challenging [1]. Stroke is considered a medical emergency, and the assumption that "time is brain" emphasizes that urgent evaluation and treatment are needed in stroke [2].

Therefore, one of the most important advantages in the management of acute cerebral disease is not pharmacological. Modifying the clinical management approach for stroke has had a beneficial impact on morbidity and mortality [3].

The greatest argument for the need to create an adequate system for the management of stroke has enabled the development of services and the creation of multidisciplinary teams: in this context, in the 21st century, stroke units were established [4].

The 1950s saw the first description of stroke unit settings for the management of stroke patients, made possible by a multidisciplinary team of stroke specialists, followed by the first trials on organized stroke rehabilitation units in the 1960s [5,6], and descriptions of intensive care stroke units in the 1970s [7].

The first large stroke unit trial was published in 1980, involving more than 300 patients [8]; in 1991, the first convincing trial demonstrated that the mortality of stroke patients was lower if they were managed in an organized setting than if they received care in general medicine or neurology departments [9].

In 1993, a meta-analysis was performed on the results of all randomized controlled trials which compared the outcomes of patients hospitalized in stroke units with those hospitalized in general departments. The authors defined a stroke unit "as incorporating a multidisciplinary team of specialists in the care of stroke patients." This definition could be used for both a stroke ward and a mobile stroke team. The review showed that care in a stroke unit setting reduced mortality by 28%, and also reduced the necessity of inpatient care, after a median of 1 year from the event [10].

The Stroke Unit Trialists' Collaboration was established with the goal of improving the results available from stroke unit trials and to update data. The Principal Investigators of all kinds of trials joined a research group. Subsequently, an updated dataset for all randomized controlled trials on stroke unit care was devised by Stroke Unit trialists' collaboration and the Cochrane group, thus confirming a reduction in mortality of 19% (over the first year), as well as reductions in disability and dependency compared with survivors [11].

The crucial point highlighted in all trials is that an expert multidisciplinary team composed of physicians, physiotherapists, nurses, and language and occupational therapists enhances patient care in a stroke unit. This trait may promote the effectiveness of stroke unit care compared with general ward care [3]. Hence, a multidisciplinary team can better manage medical complications that occur in the first week after stroke. Indeed, the difference in death rate between patients hospitalized in a stroke unit and those hospitalized in general medicine is high in the first week, when mortality is often caused by medical complications such as infections, pneumonia, etc. [3]. Furthermore, it seems that intensive physiotherapy and language therapy could improve outcomes in terms of reducing dependency [12].

In the 2000s, several observational studies showed that stroke unit care was associated with improved outcomes, and clinical practice guidelines began to recommend creating stroke units.

The World Stroke Organization has representatives from 12 countries; international guidelines to establish stroke units were redacted in 2014 [13]. This has been associated with relevant improvements in patient outcomes [14]. The Cochrane group recently confirmed this statement through a systematic review, including 5902 patients, finding moderate-quality evidence that stroke patients managed in stroke units are more likely to survive, be independent, and are less likely to require hospitalization in the first year after stroke. These results are independent of patient age, sex, stroke type, and initial stroke severity [15] (Figure 1).

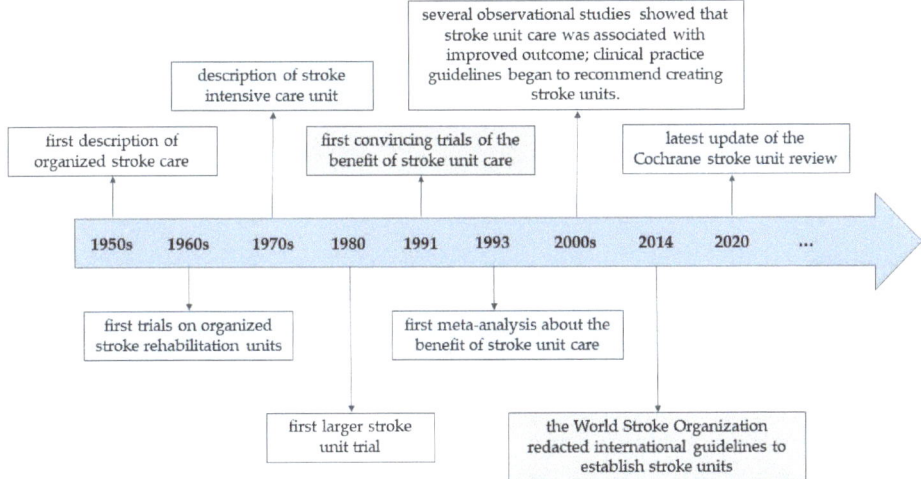

Figure 1. Milestones in the history of stroke units. Source: Authors' compilation based on data from [14].

2.2. The Stroke Registries

A stroke register is a database used for the collection of cerebrovascular-disease-related information. Over a period of substantial developments in stroke management, these registries play a crucial role as a measure of the care efficiency.

The advent of a new technological era, such as the introduction of computer systems in hospitals, has made it possible to collect data on patients with different diagnoses, including cerebrovascular diseases. Computerized databases have facilitated the collection of epidemiological data, such as possible stroke risk factors and stroke subtypes, improving clinicians' knowledge [4].

The first data collection relating to stroke management began in the 1950s, even though the term "registry" was first used in the 1970s in the context of a clinical study on stroke subtypes; subsequently, registers emerged as a central element in stroke research [16].

Over time, registers have become tools for obtaining direct feedback from clinical practice, contributing to continuous improvements in the quality of stroke care, the endorsement of innovative technologies, and the adherence to clinical guidelines by clinicians. Furthermore, the registers have also proved useful for evaluating the long-term effects of different treatments administered to an extremely heterogeneous population such as that of stroke patients [17].

Worldwide, several study projects are ongoing for the collection of data on stroke management: the comparison between participating centers is a fertile field for continuously improving clinicians' work, as well as being a useful cultural exchange.

The European Register of Stroke (EROS) project is a prospective study with the objective of estimating the impact of stroke and evaluating the quality of stroke care in European populations, analyzing the different diagnostic and therapeutic approaches [17].

In the United States, the Get With The Guidelines—Stroke program, developed by the American Heart Association/American Stroke Association (AHA/ASA), is the largest national registry for improving the quality of care and outcomes for patients affected by strokes and transient ischemic attacks (TIAs).

The use of registries has been strongly recommended by the American Heart Association to support improvements in the quality of service at the hospital level, reducing "barriers" to improving stroke care [17].

As demonstrated from data reported in the literature, we can state that in all countries where a national stroke registry has been adopted, or implemented, there has been a marked improvement in the quality of stroke care and in patient outcomes. These improvements are even more conspicuous for registries that collect patient data from hospitals all over the nation.

2.3. Challenges: The Two Side of the World

Despite all the data indicating successes in stroke unit care, there are still some key areas of challenges and uncertainties. Some components of stroke unit care remain unclear. Several trials studying early mobilization, patient positioning, infection, and glucose management have revealed contrasting results [18–21].

Despite this, the real challenge is in the management of stroke and the establishing of stroke units in low-income countries. In addition, major medical institutes in large cities are not easily accessible for many people living in rural areas.

In these settings, socioeconomic constraints lead to many patients not gaining admission to a hospital. Moreover, some of the essential components of healthcare services are lacking. A recent observational study [22] involving 108 hospitals across 28 different countries highlighted that improved outcomes are also linked to stroke unit care in low-income countries. However, the key challenge is to establish and maintain stroke units in these underdeveloped settings. Many researchers are currently trying to find low-cost protocols of care for these countries (Figure 2).

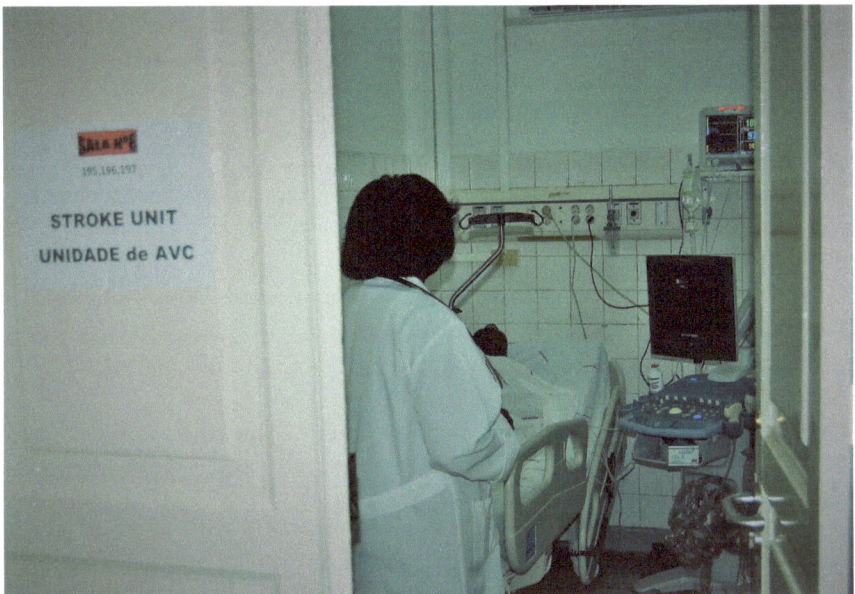

Figure 2. Stroke Unit of "Josina Machel Hospital" in Luanda, Angola. The Stroke Unit in the Neurology Department was created in 2014, led by a team of Italian Neurologists. Source: photo by author(s). Credit: © M. Paciaroni, used with permission.

3. Conclusions

Nowadays stroke units are the gold standard for acute stroke care and the development of stroke registries has facilitated the collection of clinical and epidemiological data. Nevertheless, discrepancies in stroke units management between Countries around the world is still a challenge.

Author Contributions: Conceptualization, L.G., C.C. and R.R.; writing—original draft preparation, L.G, C.C. and R.R.; writing—review and editing, L.G., C.C. and R.R.; supervision, L.G., C.C. and R.R.. All authors have read and agreed to the published version of the manuscript.

Funding: This research received no external funding.

Acknowledgments: The completion of this research project would not have been possible without the contributions and support of many colleagues. We are deeply grateful to all those who played a role in the success of this project. We would like to thank Maurizio Paciaroni for his invaluable input and support. His insights and expertise were instrumental in shaping the direction of this project.

Conflicts of Interest: The authors declare no conflict of interest.

References

1. Caplan, L.R. Caplan's short rendition of Stroke during the 20th century: Part II. *Int. J. Stroke* **2006**, *1*, 228–234. [CrossRef]
2. Saver, J.L. Time is brain—Quantified. *Stroke.* **2006**, *37*, 263–266. [CrossRef] [PubMed]

3. Sinha, S.; Warburton, E.A. The evolution of stroke units—Towards a more intensive approach? *QJM—Mon. J. Assoc. Physicians* **2000**, *93*, 633–638. [CrossRef]
4. Paciaroni, M.; Bogousslavsky, J. Chapter 1 The history of stroke and cerebrovascular disease. *Handb. Clin. Neurol.* **2008**, *92*, 3–28. [CrossRef]
5. Feldman, D.J.; Lee, P.R.; Unterecker, J.; Lloyd, K.; Rusk, H.A.; Toole, A. A comparison of functionally orientated medical care and formal rehabilitation in the management of patients with hemiplegia due to cerebrovascular disease. *J. Chronic Dis.* **1962**, *15*, 297–310. [CrossRef] [PubMed]
6. Gordon, E.E.; Kohn, K.H. Evaluation of rehabilitation methods in the hemiplegic patient. *J. Chronic Dis.* **1966**, *19*, 3–16. [CrossRef] [PubMed]
7. Millikan, C.H. Stroke intensive care units: Objectives and results. *Adv. Neurol.* **1979**, *10*, 235–237. [CrossRef]
8. Garraway, W.M.; Akhtar, A.J.; Prescott, R.J.; Hockey, L. Management of acute stroke in the elderly: Preliminary results of a controlled trial. *Br. Med. J.* **1980**, *280*, 1040–1043. [CrossRef]
9. Indredavik, B.; Bakke, F.; Solberg, R.; Rokseth, R.; Haaheim, L.L.; Holme, I. Benefit of a stroke unit: A randomized controlled trial. *Stroke* **1991**, *22*, 1026–1031. [CrossRef]
10. Langhorne, P.; Williams, B.O.; Gilchrist, W.; Howie, K. Do stroke units save lives? *Lancet* **1993**, *342*, 395–398. [CrossRef]
11. Trialists, S.U. Collaborative systematic review of the randomised trials of organised inpatient (stroke unit) care after stroke. Stroke Unit Trialists' Collaboration. *BMJ* **1997**, *314*, 1151.
12. Kwakkel, G.; Wagenaar, R.C.; Koelman, T.W.; Lankhorst, G.J.; Koetsier, J.C. Effects of intensity of rehabilitation after stroke: A research synthesis. *Stroke* **1997**, *28*, 1550–1556. [CrossRef] [PubMed]
13. Lindsay, P.; Furie, K.L.; Davis, S.M.; Donnan, G.A.; Norrving, B. World stroke organization global stroke services guidelines and action plan. *Int. J. Stroke* **2014**, *9*, 4–13. [CrossRef] [PubMed]
14. Langhorne, P. The Stroke Unit Story: Where Have We Been and Where Are We Going? *Cerebrovasc. Dis.* **2021**, *50*, 636–643. [CrossRef] [PubMed]
15. Langhorne, P.; Ramachandra, S. Organised inpatient (stroke unit) care for stroke: Network meta-analysis. *Cochrane Database Syst. Rev.* **2020**, *4*, CD000197. [CrossRef]
16. Cadilhac, D.A.; Kim, J.; Lannin, N.A.; Kapral, M.K.; Schwamm, L.H.; Dennis, M.S.; Norrving, B.; Meretoja, A. National stroke registries for monitoring and improving the quality of hospital care: A systematic review. *Int. J. Stroke* **2016**, *11*, 28–40. [CrossRef]
17. Tanne, D.; Koton, S.; Bornstein, N.M. National Stroke Registries: What can we learn from them? *Neurology* **2013**, *81*, 1257–1259. [CrossRef]
18. Bernhardt, J.; Langhorne, P.; Lindley, R.I.; Thrift, A.G.; Ellery, F.; Collier, J.; Churilov, L.; Moodie, M.; Dewey, H.; Donnan, G. Efficacy and safety of very early mobilisation within 24 h of stroke onset (AVERT): A randomised controlled trial. *Lancet* **2017**. Erratum in *Lancet* **2015**, *386*, 46–55. [CrossRef]
19. Anderson, C.S.; Arima, H.; Lavados, P.; Billot, L.; Hackett, M.L.; Olavarría, V.V.; Venturelli, P.M.; Brunser, A.; Peng, B.; Cui, L.; et al. Cluster-Randomized, Crossover Trial of Head Positioning in Acute Stroke. *N. Engl. J. Med.* **2017**, *376*, 2437–2447. [CrossRef]

20. Middleton, S.; McElduff, P.; Ward, J.; Grimshaw, J.M.; Dale, S.; D'Este, C.; Drury, P.; Griffiths, R.; Cheung, N.W.; Quinn, C.; et al. Implementation of evidence-based treatment protocols to manage fever, hyperglycaemia, and swallowing dysfunction in acute stroke (QASC): A cluster randomised controlled trial. *Lancet* **2011**, *378*, 1699–1706. [CrossRef]
21. Vermeij, J.D.; Westendorp, W.F.; Dippel, D.W.J.; van de Beek, D.; Nederkoorn, P.J. Antibiotic therapy for preventing infections in people with acute stroke. *Cochrane Database Syst. Rev.* **2018**, *2018*, CD008530. [CrossRef]
22. Langhorne, P.; O'Donnell, M.J.; Chin, S.L.; Zhang, H.; Xavier, D.; Avezum, A.; Mathur, N.; Turner, M.; MacLeod, M.J.; Lopez-Jaramillo, P.; et al. Practice patterns and outcomes after stroke across countries at different economic levels (INTERSTROKE): An international observational study. *Lancet* **2018**, *391*, 2019–2027. [CrossRef] [PubMed]

© 2023 by the authors. Licensee MDPI, Basel, Switzerland. This article is an open access article distributed under the terms and conditions of the Creative Commons Attribution (CC BY) license (http://creativecommons.org/licenses/by/4.0/).

From Thrombolysis, to Thrombectomy in Acute Ischemic Stroke

Norbert Nighoghossian

Abstract: Until the early 1990s, ischemic stroke (IS) was considered a sinister fatality due to a lack of effective recanalization therapy allowing a prompt reperfusion of the ischemic brain, a key factor in reducing neurological disability. Over the past 30 years, the ischemic penumbra has gradually become the target of new reperfusion strategies to reduce ischemic stroke-related neurological disability. Ischemic stroke therapy has benefited from three major advances that upset its management: (1) The benefit of intravenous thrombolysis by Tissue Plasminogen Activator rt-PA. (2) The success of endovascular treatment for large arteries occlusion. (3) The development of stroke imaging. The "time is brain" aphorism anchored IS in the emergency field, which led to rapid transfers to stroke units. We propose to report the main stages of this therapeutic transformation in this major area of public health. Although access to these transformations remains limited in the world and much remains to be done to improve the IS care system, this area has experienced an unprecedented upheaval in the history of neurology.

1. Introduction

Until the early 1990s, ischemic stroke was marked by fate and a mere object of curiosity for neurologists fond of anatomoclinic confrontations. Despite the advances related to the discovery of the ischemic penumbra concept by Astrup [1], patients languished in emergency departments without brain imaging to differentiate between IS or hemorrhagic stroke. This approach was justified for many doctors by the lack of effective recanalization therapy restoring the brain blood flow. However, during the last 30 years, this pathology would benefit from major therapeutic transformations that upset its management and reduce the burden of IS disability. This upheaval lies in two dates: 1995, with the validation of rtPA in acute ischemic stroke in the United States, and 2015, with the approval of thrombectomy for large artery occlusion [2]. In addition, advances in stroke brain imaging have made it possible to better identify the area at risk of infarction whose salvage is the key to reducing neurological disability. As a result, the "time is brain" aphorism anchored IS in the emergency field and has allowed prompt transfer to stroke units. In fact stroke management became very close to myocardial infarction management as IS care has clearly integrated the validated therapeutics in cardiology developed 20 years earlier.

2. Literature Review

2.1. The Penumbra Concept

The penumbra is an unstable dynamic area that circumscribes the ischemic core [1], and its preservation is essential to limit the extent of ischemic damage and subsequent disability. The ischemic penumbra should be considered as a target for reperfusion and neuroprotective treatments.

2.2. Dicovery of Thrombolytics and First Application

The discovery of thrombolytics dates back to the 1930s [3,4]. Although effective in patients with peripheral arteries, these agents such as streptokinase or urokinase were not intended to treat ischemic stroke clots [5]. In 1958, Sussman and Fitch [6] reported the first use in AIS. Overall, early studies of thrombolytic therapy have been associated with disastrous results in the absence of relevant technical conditions and imaging tools to distinguish between ischemic and hemorrhagic stroke, and even pilot studies using angiography were struck by the same degree of inefficacity. However, computed tomography (CT) was not available at this time; accordingly, the distinction between hemorrhagic and ischemic stroke was not possible. In addition, clinical trials with streptokinase in the 1990s failed [7–9]. Some of these failures might be related to the lack of a real stroke network and poor stroke expertise in several countries and likely to an increased therapeutic time window and a higher risk of molecule-specific bleeding.

2.3. Efficacy of Second Generation Drugs in AIS: Intravenous Tissue Plasminogen Activator (rt-PA)

In 1979, the discovery of tissue-type plasminogen activator (t-PA) by Désiré, Baron Collen. Refs. [10,11] would disrupt the therapeutic field of ischemic stroke.

2.4. rt-PA, the First Experimental Approach in IS

The experimental work of Justin Zivin on a thrombo-embolic stroke model in rabbit showed that r-tPA improved neurological status [12]. Thus, this work paved the way to clinical trials.

2.5. Clinical Trials of rt-PA in IS

Tom Brott, Clarke Haley and David Levy developed the first stroke network [13] dedicated to the treatment of the IS by rt-PA. The positive results of NINDS rt-PA stroke study trial led to the approval of *rt-PA* in the USA within 3 h of onset of symptoms in 1995 [2].

2.6. The Lazarus Effect

The unprecedented clinical recovery following this treatment was compared to the resurrection of Lazarus, the greatest miracle accomplished by Jesus. Despite this effect of r-tPA in IS and the fact that neurologists may dramatically change the world's approach of IS, the NINDS studies were the matter of severe controversy.

2.7. What Happened in Europe During This Time?

During the same period, there was a duel between supporters of rt-PA led by a hero of German vascular neurology, Professor Werner Hacke, and those of streptokinase led by Professor Hommel. Throughout the studies, the t-PA came out the winner of this confrontation, which lasted at least 7 years. Approval of rt-PA required a set of clinical trials involving varying doses and delivery times [14,15].

The pooled analysis of six randomized trials [16] showed that early administration of t-PA was associated with a better outcome, thus t-PA was definitively approved only in 2003 in Europe. The ECASS3 trial also initiated by Werner Hacke allowed successively lengthening the therapeutic window at 4H30 [17,18]. However, alteplase still remained underused; less than 10% of patients receive this treatment in most countries.

2.8. Intravenous Tissue Plasminogen Activator t-PA for Wake Up Stroke

Until 2015, due to the unknown time of symptom onset, patients with wake-up or without witness stroke were not treated by T-PA [19], although wake-up stroke accounted for almost 20% of ischemic stroke [20,21]. A German neurologist, Pr Götz Thomalla from the University Medical Center Hamburg—Eppendorf, suggested that the mismatch between a visible acute ischemic lesion on DWI and the absence of marked parenchymal hyperintensity on fluid-attenuated inversion recovery (FLAIR) images (DWI–FLAIR mismatch) may likely identify an ischemic stroke that occurred within 4.5 h of stroke onset [22]. As a result, the WAKE-UP trial showed that rT-PA was effective in patients with such imaging patterns [23].

2.9. Intravenous Tissue Plasminogen Activator t-PA Treatment between 4.5 and 9 h after Known Onset with the Use of Advanced Imaging

The introduction of perfusion imaging methods (CT/MRI) allowed patients to be treated in a later time window due to a better analysis of tissue at risk of infarction [24]. In patients who were imaged with CT perfusion or perfusion-diffusion MRI, within 4.5–9 h, a meta-analysis has shown that thrombolysis with rT-PA improves the neurological outcome [25].

3. Mechanical Thrombectomy: A Breakthrough Therapy in IS Treatment. Overview of Thrombectomy Trials

Most people with large artery occlusion fared poorly with *rt-PA*. Although previous trials published in 2013 were associated with negative outcomes, [26–28], further studies documented the benefit of thrombectomys within 6 hours from symptom onset [29–37]. These results were likely related to a better patient selection, shorter door-to-arterial access times and improvement of devices.

3.1. Endovascular Treatment Up to 16 or 24 h

Recently the time window for mechanical thrombectomy was extended up to 16 or 24 h if advanced stroke imaging identify a salvageable penumbra. Therefore, current guidelines recommend thrombectomy in the 6- to 24-hour time window for patients meeting these imaging criteria [38,39].

4. Thrombectomy Some Outstanding Issues

4.1. Thrombectomy in Minor IS

The benefit of thrombectomy in patients presenting with anterior circulation LVO and minor stroke is still debated [40]. However, a substantial proportion of minor strokes are subsequently disabled at 90 days [41,42]. Patients with minor strokes and proximal occlusions may experience clinical deterioration due to collateral failure if not promptly recanalized [43], especially since thrombectomy for minor stroke patient (NIHSS ≤ 5) seems effective [44].

4.2. Thrombectomy for Distal Occlusion

The benefit of thrombectomy in patients with distal occlusion is less obvious [45]. However, some observational data have suggested a potential benefit in proximal M2. Accordingly, further research are needed to confirm the benefit of thrombectomy in distal M2 occlusion and even in anterior or posterior cerebral artery occlusion.

4.3. Thrombectomy for Large Core Volume

Large core volume is associated with severe disability [46]. Several randomized controlled trials have recently confirmed the potential benefit of mechanical thrombectomy regardless of the initial core volume.

4.4. Thrombectomy for Basilar Artery Occlusion

Since the masterful description of Kubik and Adams [47] basilar artery occlusion remained a therapeutic challenge. Attempts at intra-arterial thrombolytic treatments gave rise to some hope in the 1990s [48]. More recently, clinical trials demonstrated lower rates of death and an improved modified Rankin scale with thrombectomy as compared to the best medical management [49–51].

4.5. Direct Thrombectomy Versus Standard of Care

The DIRECT-MT study (Direct endovascular thrombectomy with or without Intravenous Alteplase in Acute Stroke) [52] found similar results between direct thrombectomy and combined thrombolysis–thrombectomy arms; however, further studies are needed to validate this approach.

5. Pathway Design for IS Care in the Era of Endovascular Thrombectomy

Although the effectiveness of thrombectomy is clearly validated, the eligibility is still poor. Treatment delivery depends on the existing local network. Currently, there are two models; first, the drip-and-ship model entails initial routing of patients to the nearest primary stroke center (PSC) for diagnostic work-up and IVT. Subsequently, patients may be transported to the nearest comprehensive stroke center (CSC) to undergo EVT. Secondly, the mothership model, where patients are routed directly to a CSC for IVT administration and, if appropriate, mechanical thrombectomy.

5.1. Prehospital Triage

Several prehospital triage tools have been proposed to distinguish patients with proximal occlusion from distal occlusion. Four prehospital triage tools to detect or predict LVO can be distinguished: prehospital triage scales, telemedicine supported triage, on site computed tomography (CT)-angiography, and some experimental noninvasive tools [53–56]. However, currently they are no prehospital triage scales available with acceptable sensitivity and specificity [57].

The inclusion of CT and CT-angiography in mobile stroke units (MSUs) may establish on site the distinction between LVO and non-LVO . MSUs may shorten the time to treatment both for IVT and EVT, which has been proven [58].

5.2. The Main Limitation for Thrombecctomy is the Low Number of Interventional Neuroradiology Specialists a Call for the Decompartmentalization of Specialties for the Same Purpose: the Prompt Reperfusion of the Ischemic Brain

The main limitation for thrombectomy is the low number of interventional neuroradiology specialists compared to what is observed in cardiology. We need to increase the number of physicians trained for this task, thus increasing the eligibility to thrombectomy. Indeed, we now face an overwhelming shortage of neurointerventionists that may compromise IS treatment. Therefore, other physicians trained in neurointerventional procedures must now fill this gap in AIS, in order to increase patients eligibility for mechanical thrombectomy.

6. Conclusions

This review highlighted the major transformations over the past 30 years in ischemic stroke therapy. The road is still long to increase access to optimpal stroke care, but the tools exist, and our main fault would be not to use them more effectively to reduce the handicap of a condition that we have stored for years in the locker room of fatality.

Conflicts of Interest: The authors declare no conflict of interest.

References

1. Astrup, J.; Symon, L.; Branston, N.M.; Lassen, N.A. Cortical evoked potential and extracellular K+ and H+ at critical levels of brain ischemia. *Stroke* **1977**, *8*, 51–57. [CrossRef]
2. NINDS tPA Study Group. Tissue plasminogen activator for acute ischemic stroke. *N. Engl. J. Med.* **1995**, *333*, 1581–1587. [CrossRef]
3. Tillett, W.S.; Garner, R.L. The fibrinolytic activity of hemolytic streptococci. *J. Exp. Med.* **1933**, *58*, 485–502. [CrossRef]
4. Tillett, W.S.; Johnson, A.J.; McCarty, W.R. The intravenous infusion of the streptococcal fibrinolytic Principle (streptokinase) into patients. *J. Clin. Investig.* **1955**, *34*, 169–185. [CrossRef]
5. Macfarlane, R.G.; Pilling, J. Fibrinolytic activity of normal urine. *Nature* **1947**, *159*, 779. [CrossRef]
6. Sussman, B.J.; Fitch, T.S. Thrombolysis with fibrinolysin in cerebral arterial occlusion. *JAMA* **1958**, *167*, 1705–1709. [CrossRef]
7. Trial—Italy, Multicentre Acute Stroke. Randomised controlled trial of streptokinase, aspirin, and combination of both in treatment of acute ischaemic stroke: Multicentre Acute Stroke Trial—Italy (MAST-I) Group. *Lancet* **1995**, *346*, 1509–1514. [CrossRef]
8. Multicenter Acute Stroke Trial—Europe Study Group. Thrombolytic therapy with streptokinase in acute ischemic stroke: Multicenter Acute Stroke Trial—Europe study group. *N. Engl. J. Med.* **1996**, *335*, 145–150. [CrossRef]
9. Fujishima, M.; Omae, T.; Tanaka, K.; Iino, K.; Matsuo, O.; Mihara, H. Controlled trial of combined urokinase and dextran sulfate therapy in patients with acute cerebral infarction. *Angiology* **1986**, *37*, 487–498. [CrossRef]
10. Rijken, D.C.; Collen, D. Purification and characterization of the plasminogen activator secreted by human melanoma cells in culture. *J. Biol. Chem.* **1981**, *256*, 7035–7041. [CrossRef]
11. Collen, D.; Lijnen, H.R. Tissue-type plasminogen activator: A historical perspective and personal account. *J. Thromb. Haemost.* **2004**, *2*, 541–546. [CrossRef]
12. Zivin, J.A.; Fisher, M.; DeGirolami, U.; Hemenway, C.C.; Stashak, J.A. Tissue plasminogen activator reduces neurological damage after cerebral embolism. *Science* **1985**, *230*, 1289–1292. [CrossRef]
13. Brott, T.G.; Haley, E.C.; Levy, D.E.; Barsan, W.; Broderick, J.; Sheppard, G.L.; Spilker, J.; Kongable, G.L.; Massey, S.; Reed, R. Urgent therapy for stroke. Part I. Pilot study of tissue plasminogen activator administered within 90 minutes. *Stroke* **1992**, *23*, 632–640. [CrossRef]
14. Hacke, W.; Kaste, M.; Fieschi, C.; Toni, D.; Lesaffre, E.; Von Kummer, R.; Boysen, G.; Bluhmki, E.; Höxter, G.; Mahagne, M.-H.; et al. Intravenous thrombolysis with recombinant tissue plasminogen activator for acute hemispheric stroke: The European Cooperative Acute Stroke Study (ECASS). *JAMA* **1995**, *274*, 1017–1025. [CrossRef]
15. Hacke, W.; Kaste, M.; Fieschi, C.; Von Kummer, R.; Davalos, A.; Meier, D.; Larrue, V.; Bluhmki, E.; Davis, S.; Donnan, G.; et al. Randomised double-blind placebo-controlled trial of thrombolytic therapy with intravenous alteplase in acute ischaemic stroke (ECASS II). *Lancet* **1998**, *352*, 1245–1251. [CrossRef]

16. Hacke, W.; Donnan, G.; Fieschi, C.; the ATLANTIS Trials Investigators; the ECASS Trials Investigators; the NINDS rt-PA Study Group Investigators. Association of outcome with early stroke treatment: Pooled analysis of ATLANTIS, ECASS, and NINDS rt-PA stroke trials. *Lancet* **2004**, *363*, 768–774.
17. Hacke, W.; Kaste, M.; Bluhmki, E.; the ECASS Investigators. Thrombolysis with alteplase 3 to 4·5 hours after acute ischemic stroke. *N. Engl. J. Med.* **2008**, *359*, 1317–1329. [CrossRef]
18. Emberson, J.; Lees, K.R.; Lyden, P.; Blackwell, L.; Albers, G.; Bluhmki, E.; Brott, T.; Cohen, G.; Davis, S.; Donnan, G.; et al. Effect of treatment delay, age, and stroke severity on the effects of intravenous thrombolysis with alteplase for acute ischaemic stroke: A meta-analysis of individualpatient data from randomised trials. *Lancet* **2014**, *384*, 1929–1935. [CrossRef]
19. Mackey, J.; Kleindorfer, D.; Sucharew, H.; Moomaw, C.J.; Kissela, B.M.; Alwell, K.; Flaherty, M.L.; Woo, D.; Khatri, P.; Adeoye, O.; et al. Population-based study of wake-up strokes. *Neurology* **2011**, *76*, 1662–1667. [CrossRef]
20. Reid, J.M.; Dai, D.; Cheripelli, B.; Christian, C.; Reidy, Y.; Gubitz, G.J.; Phillips, S.J. Differences in wake-up and unknown onset stroke examined in a stroke registry. *Int. J. Stroke* **2015**, *10*, 331–335. [CrossRef]
21. Thomalla, G.; Cheng, B.; Ebinger, M.; Hao, Q.; Tourdias, T.; Wu, O.; Kim, J.S.; Breuer, L.; Singer, O.C.; Warach, S.; et al. DWI-FLAIR mismatch for the identification of patients with acute ischaemic stroke within 4.5 h of symptom onset (PRE-FLAIR): A multicentre observational study. *Lancet Neurol.* **2011**, *10*, 978–986. [CrossRef]
22. Thomalla, G.; Simonsen, C.Z.; Boutitie, F.; Andersen, G.; Berthezene, Y.; Cheng, B.; Cheripelli, B.; Cho, T.-H.; Fazekas, F.; Fiehler, J.; et al. MRI-guided thrombolysis for stroke with unknown time of onset. *N. Engl. J. Med.* **2018**, *379*, 611–622. [CrossRef]
23. Ma, H.; Campbell, B.C.V.; Parsons, M.W.; Churilov, L.; Levi, C.R.; Hsu, C.; Kleinig, T.J.; Wijeratne, T.; Curtze, S.; Dewey, H.M.; et al. Thrombolysis guided by perfusion imaging up to 9 hours after onset of stroke. *N. Engl. J. Med.* **2019**, *380*, 1795–1803. [CrossRef]
24. Campbell, B.C.V.; Ma, H.; Ringleb, P.A.; Parsons, M.; Churilov, L.; Bendszus, M.; Levi, C.; Hsu, C.; Kleinig, T.; Fatar, M. Extending thrombolysis to 4.5-9 h and wake-up stroke using perfusion imaging: A systematic review and meta-analysis of individual patient data. *Lancet* **2019**, *394*, 139–147. [CrossRef]
25. Broderick, J.P.; Palesch, Y.Y.; Demchuk, A.M.; Yeatts, S.D.; Khatri, P.; Hill, M.D.; Jauch, E.C.; Jovin, T.G.; Yan, B.; Silver, F.L.; et al. Endovascular therapy after intravenous t-PA versus t-PA alone for stroke. *N. Engl. J. Med.* **2013**, *368*, 893–903. [CrossRef]
26. Ciccone, A.; Valvassori, L.; Nichelatti, M.; Sgoifo, A.; Ponzio, M.; Sterzi, R.; Boccardi, E. Endovascular treatment for acute ischemic stroke. *N. Engl. J. Med.* **2013**, *368*, 904–913. [CrossRef]
27. Kidwell, C.S.; Jahan, R.; Gornbein, J.; Alger, J.R.; Nenov, V.; Ajani, Z.; Feng, L.; Meyer, B.C.; Olson, S.; Schwamm, L.H.; et al. A trial of imaging selection and endovascular treatment for ischemic stroke. *N. Engl. J. Med.* **2013**, *368*, 914–923. [CrossRef]
28. Berkhemer, O.A.; Fransen, P.S.; Beumer, D.; van den Berg, L.A.; Lingsma, H.F.; Yoo, A.J.; Schonewille, W.J.; Vos, J.A.; Nederkoorn, P.J.; Wermer, M.J.H.; et al. A randomized trial of intraarterial treatment for acute ischemic stroke. *N. Engl. J. Med.* **2015**, *372*, 11–20. [CrossRef]

29. Campbell, B.C.; Mitchell, P.J.; Kleinig, T.J.; Dewey, H.M.; Churilov, L.; Yassi, N.; Yan, B.; Dowling, R.J.; Parsons, M.W.; Oxley, T.J.; et al. Endovascular therapy for ischemic stroke with perfusion-imaging selection. *N. Engl. J. Med.* **2015**, *372*, 1009–1018. [CrossRef]
30. Goyal, M.; Demchuk, A.M.; Menon, B.K.; Eesa, M.; Rempel, J.L.; Thornton, J.; Roy, D.; Jovin, T.G.; Willinsky, R.A.; Sapkota, B.L.; et al. Randomized assessment of rapid endovascular treatment of ischemic stroke. *N. Engl. J. Med.* **2015**, *372*, 1019–1030. [CrossRef]
31. Saver, J.L.; Goyal, M.; Bonafe, A.; Diener, H.C.; Levy, E.I.; Pereira, V.M.; Albers, G.W.; Cognard, C.; Cohen, D.J.; Hacke, W.; et al. Stent retriever thrombectomy after intravenous t-PA vs. t-PA alone in stroke. *N. Engl. J. Med.* **2015**, *372*, 2285–2295. [CrossRef]
32. Jovin, T.G.; Chamorro, A.; Cobo, E.; de Miquel, M.A.; Molina, C.A.; Rovira, A.; Román, L.S.; Serena, J.; Abilleira, S.; Ribó, M.; et al. Thrombectomy within 8 hours after symptom onset in ischemic stroke. *N. Engl. J. Med.* **2015**, *372*, 2296–2306. [CrossRef]
33. Bracard, S.; Ducrocq, X.; Mas, J.L.; Soudant, M.; Oppenheim, C.; Moulin, T.; Guillemin, F.; THRACE investigators. Mechanical thrombectomy after intravenous alteplase versus alteplase alone after stroke (THRACE): A randomised controlled trial. *Lancet Neurol.* **2016**, *15*, 1138–1147. [CrossRef]
34. Goyal, M.; Menon, B.K.; van Zwam, W.H.; Dippel, D.W.; Mitchell, P.J.; Demchuk, A.M.; Dávalos, A.; Majoie, C.B.L.M.; van der Lugt, A.; de Miquel, M.A.; et al. Endovascular thrombectomy after large-vessel ischaemic stroke: A meta-analysis of individual patient data from five randomised trials. *Lancet* **2016**, *387*, 1723–1731. [CrossRef]
35. Saver, J.L.; Goyal, M.; van der Lugt, A.; Menon, B.K.; Majoie, C.B.; Dippel, D.W.; Campbell, B.C.; Nogueira, R.G.; Demchuk, A.M.; Tomasello, A.; et al. Time to treatment with endovascular thrombectomy and outcomes from ischemic stroke: A meta-analysis. *JAMA* **2016**, *316*, 1279–1288. [CrossRef] [PubMed]
36. Campbell, B.C.V.; De Silva, D.A.; Macleod, M.R.; Coutts, S.B.; Schwamm, L.H.; Davis, S.M.; Donnan, G.A. Ischaemic stroke. *Nat. Rev. Dis. Prim.* **2019**, *5*, 70. [CrossRef]
37. Albers, G.W.; Marks, M.P.; Kemp, S.; Christensen, S.; Tsai, J.P.; Ortega-Gutierrez, S.; McTaggart, R.A.; Torbey, M.T.; Kim-Tenser, M.; Leslie-Mazwi, T.; et al. Thrombectomy for stroke at 6 to 16 hours with selection by perfusion imaging. *N. Engl. J. Med.* **2018**, *378*, 708–718. [CrossRef]
38. Nogueira, R.G.; Jadhav, A.P.; Haussen, D.C.; Bonafe, A.; Budzik, R.F.; Bhuva, P.; Yavagal, D.R.; Ribo, M.; Cognard, C.; Hanel, R.A.; et al. Thrombectomy 6 to 24 hours after stroke with a mismatch between deficit and infarct. *N. Engl. J. Med.* **2018**, *378*, 11–21. [CrossRef]
39. Nagel, S.; Bouslama, M.; Krause, L.U.; Küpper, C.; Messer, M.; Petersen, M.; Lowens, S.; Herzberg, M.; Ringleb, P.A.; Möhlenbruch, M.A.; et al. Mechanical thrombectomy in patients with milder strokes and large vessel occlusions. *Stroke* **2018**, *49*, 2391–2397. [CrossRef]
40. Khatri, P.; Conaway, M.R.; Johnston, K.C.; Acute Stroke Accurate Prediction Study (ASAP) Investigators. Ninety-day outcome rates of a prospective cohort of consecutive patients with mild ischemic stroke. *Stroke* **2012**, *43*, 560–562. [CrossRef]

41. Haussen, D.C.; Bouslama, M.; Grossberg, J.A.; Anderson, A.; Belagage, S.; Frankel, M.; Bianchi, N.; Rebello, L.C.; Nogueira, R.G. Too good to intervene? Thrombectomy for large vessel occlusion strokes with minimal symptoms: An intention-to-treat analysis. *J. Neurointerv. Surg.* **2017**, *9*, 917–921. [CrossRef]
42. Campbell, B.C.; Christensen, S.; Tress, B.M.; Churilov, L.; Desmond, P.M.; Parsons, M.W.; Barber, P.A.; Levi, C.; Bladin, C.; Donnan, G.; et al. Failure of collateral blood flow is associated with infarct growth in ischemic stroke. *J. Cereb. Blood Flow Metab.* **2013**, *33*, 1168–1172. [CrossRef] [PubMed]
43. Menon, B.K.; Hill, M.D.; Davalos, A.; Roos, Y.B.W.E.M.; Campbell, B.C.V.; Dippel, D.W.J.; Guillemin, F.; Saver, J.L.; van der Lugt, A.; Demchuk, A.M.; et al. Efficacy of endovascular thrombectomy in patients with M2 segment middle cerebral artery occlusions: Meta-analysis of data from the HERMES Collaboration. *J. Neurointerv. Surg.* **2019**, *11*, 1065–1069. [CrossRef] [PubMed]
44. Rebello, L.C.; Bouslama, M.; Haussen, D.C.; Dehkharghani, S.; Grossberg, J.A.; Belagaje, S.; Frankel, M.R.; Nogueira, R.G. Endovascular treatment for patients with acute stroke who have a large ischemic core and large mismatch imaging profile. *JAMA Neurol.* **2017**, *74*, 34–40. [CrossRef] [PubMed]
45. Campbell, B.C.V.; Majoie, C.B.L.M.; Albers, G.W.; Menon, B.K.; Yassi, N.; Sharma, G.; van Zwam, W.H.; van Oostenbrugge, R.J.; Demchuk, A.M.; Guillemin, F.; et al. Penumbral imaging and functional outcome in patients with anterior circulation ischaemic stroke treated with endovascular thrombectomy versus medical therapy: A meta-analysis of individual patient-level data. *Lancet Neurol.* **2019**, *18*, 46–55. [CrossRef] [PubMed]
46. Kubik, C.S.; Adams, R.D. Occlusion of the basilar artery—A clinical and pathologic study. *Brain* **1946**, *69*, 73–121. [CrossRef]
47. Hacke, W.; Zeumer, H.; Ferbert, A.; Brückmann, H.; del Zoppo, G.J. Intra-arterial thrombolytic therapy improves outcome in patients with acute vertebrobasilar occlusive disease. *Stroke* **1988**, *19*, 1216–1222. [CrossRef]
48. Kumar, G.; Shahripour, R.B.; Alexandrov, A.V. Recanalization of acute basilar artery occlusion improves outcomes: A meta-analysis. *J. Neurointerv. Surg.* **2015**, *7*, 868–874. [CrossRef]
49. Liu, X.; Dai, Q.; Ye, R.; Zi, W.; Liu, Y.; Wang, H.; Zhu, W.; Ma, M.; Yin, Q.; Li, M.; et al. Endovascular treatment versus standard medical treatment for vertebrobasilar artery occlusion (BEST): An open-label, randomised controlled trial. *Lancet Neurol.* **2020**, *19*, 115–122. [CrossRef]
50. Schonewille, W. BASICS—A Randomized Acute Stroke Trial of Endovascular Therapy in Acute Basilar Artery Occlusion. European Stroke. Organisation Conference 2020 Large Clinical Trials—Webinar. Available online: https://eso-wso-conference.org/eso-wso-may-webinar/ (accessed on 12 November 2020).
51. Demaerschalk, B.M.; Berg, J.; Chong, B.W.; Gross, H.; Nystrom, K.; Adeoye, O.; Schwamm, L.; Wechsler, L.; Whitchurch, S. American telemedicine association: Telestroke guidelines. *Telemed J. E Health* **2017**, *23*, 376–389. [CrossRef]
52. Thorpe, S.G.; Thibeault, C.M.; Canac, N.; Wilk, S.J.; Devlin, T.; Hamilton, R.B. Decision criteria for large vessel occlusion using transcranial doppler waveform morphology. *Front. Neurol.* **2018**, *9*, 847. [CrossRef] [PubMed]

53. Kellner, C.P.; Sauvageau, E.; Snyder, K.V.; Fargen, K.M.; Arthur, A.S.; Turner, R.D.; Alexandrov, A.V. The VITAL study and overall pooled analysis with the VIPS non-invasive stroke detection device. *J. Neurointerv. Surg.* **2018**, *10*, 1079–1084. [CrossRef]
54. Krebs, W.; Sharkey-Toppen, T.P.; Cheek, F.; Cortez, E.; Larrimore, A.; Keseg, D.; Panchal, A.R. Prehospital stroke assessment for large vessel occlusions: A systematic review. *Prehosp. Emerg. Care* **2018**, *22*, 180–188. [CrossRef] [PubMed]
55. John, S.; Stock, S.; Masaryk, T.; Bauer, A.; Cerejo, R.; Uchino, K.; Winners, S.; Rasmussen, P.; Hussain, M.S. Performance of CT angiography on a mobile stroke treatment unit: Implications for triage. *J. Neuroimaging* **2016**, *26*, 391–394. [CrossRef] [PubMed]
56. Czap, A.L.; Singh, N.; Bowry, R.; Jagolino-Cole, A.; Parker, S.A.; Phan, K.; Wang, M.; Sheth, S.A.; Rajan, S.S.; Yamal, J.M.; et al. Mobile stroke unit computed tomography angiography substantially shortens door-to-puncture time. *Stroke* **2020**, *51*, 1613–1615. [CrossRef]
57. Fatima, N.; Saqqur, M.; Hussain, M.S.; Shuaib, A. Mobile stroke unit versus standard medical care in the management of patients with acute stroke: A systematic review and meta-analysis. *Int. J. Stroke* **2020**, *15*, 595–608. [CrossRef]
58. Kim, J.; Easton, D.; Zhao, H.; Coote, S.; Sookram, G.; Smith, K.; Stephenson, M.; Bernard, S.; Parsons, M.; Yan, B.; et al. Economic evaluation of the Melbourne Mobile Stroke Unit. *Int. J. Stroke* **2021**, *16*, 466–475. [CrossRef]

© 2023 by the author. Licensee MDPI, Basel, Switzerland. This article is an open access article distributed under the terms and conditions of the Creative Commons Attribution (CC BY) license (http://creativecommons.org/licenses/by/4.0/).

The History of Clinical Neuroprotection Failure

Lucia Gentili, Carmen Calvello and Roberta Rinaldi

Abstract: Neuroprotection in stroke treatment refers to a group of treatments and drugs aimed to antagonize the biochemical and molecular processes that lead to irreversible ischemic damage. In recent years, several clinical studies have been conducted to test the efficacy of several promising molecules with different mechanisms of action. However, the results obtained from preclinical studies (on in vitro models or on animals), despite having provided excellent results, making the goal of stroke neuroprotection at least achievable, were accompanied by a high failure rate. The reasons for these failures are linked to the unbridgeable difference between the animal and human models and to the marked heterogeneity of stroke in humans. Although future perspectives are encouraging, other techniques such as neuroprotectant cocktails, reperfusion, improving angiogenesis and collateral circulations, and infarction prevention, may represent a goal in stroke neuroprotection.

1. Neuroprotection in Stroke: Number of Molecules from Past to Present

Over the past 30 years, further research in the field of neuroprotection has been conducted. Neuroprotection could be defined as any strategy applied to antagonize molecular and cellular events that lead to ischemia, targeting brain cells to improve their survival [1].

First studies emerged from the 1970s, but the crucial development occurred in the 1990s and 2000s when the basis of ischemic damage was discovered. Excitotoxicity, caused by a reduction in blood flow, was the first mechanism of brain injury, which helped the comprehension of many underlying processes and the detection of relevant therapeutic targets for ischemic stroke [2]. There was a growing sense that ischemic stroke was not only a vascular disease, but many vascular and neural cells such as astrocytes, macrophages, neurons, and endothelial cells formed a unique entity involved in the damage [3]. These results suggest that brain injury was not only the product of local alteration, but many systemic mechanisms could be also involved [4].

Magnesium sulfate acts as a neuroprotector in the middle cerebral artery occlusion model in rodents, blocking the N-methyl-D-aspartate (NMDA) receptors, reducing glutamate release, and blocking calcium channels [5]. In 2004, a large multicenter randomized controlled trial (RCT) on the intravenous infusion of magnesium did not report any benefit; this was attributed to a delay in the administration of molecules (after 12 h from acute brain injury). In 2014, another multicenter, randomized, double-blind, placebo vs controlled pivotal phase III trial (FAST_MAG) studied the administration of magnesium in patients within 2 hours after stroke; thus, magnesium treatment was inferior to the placebo (Table 1).

Antioxidant oxidative stress is one of the main mechanisms implicated in ischemic injury. Reactive oxygen species (ROS) scavengers have shown neuroprotective effects in preclinical models [6], even if these results have not been confirmed in clinical studies. Data on ebselen are contrasting; in a few studies [7,8], it seems to reduce brain injury due to cerebral ischemia, and RCT shows that receiving ebselen within 6 h from the event reduces the infarction and improves the functional outcome [9]. Unfortunately, a recent phase III trial did not confirm the neuroprotective action of this molecule [10]. Following the high-quality evidence shown in preclinical studies, a Cochrane review in 2011 [11] highlighted the inefficacy of edaravone. However, in 2013, a clinical study showed the efficacy of edaravone administered in combination with thrombolysis, increasing the revascularization and reducing the infarction of the lesion [12] (Table 1).

Haematopoietic growth factor: Granulocyte-colony-stimulating factor (G-CSF) and erythropoietin (EPO) reduce the excitotoxicity induced by glutamate, and also increase the neuroangiogenesis with an anti-inflammatory and anti-apoptotic action. G-CSF appears to be neuroprotective in preclinical studies where it seems to reduce the infarct size and the functional outcome [13,14]. These results are confirmed, even if the administration is delayed within 72 h [15]. Regardless, clinical trials are discouraging. In a multicenter RCT (AX200), the EV administration of G-CSF within 72 h did not lead to better outcomes compared to the placebo, in terms of NIHSS scores and mRS [16]. Likewise, a Cochrane review of 8 RCTs showed that G-CSF did not improve functional outcomes [17]. With regards to EPO, animal stroke models have pointed out the efficacy of this molecule in reducing infarction [18,19]. Clinically, RCT showed an increased risk of infarction and mortality in patients treated with EPO and r-tPA in combination [20] (Table 1).

Statins molecules, at high doses, have a neuroprotective effect in ischemic brain injury, thus improving endothelial function, vasodilatation, and antithrombotic and anti-inflammatory effects [21]. It is already known that the pre-stroke administration of statin has a functional benefit, even if the administration in combination with tPA seems to increase the risk of infarction [22]. Post-stroke statin therapy in naive patients within 72 h from acute event did not improve outcomes, as confirmed by RCTs [23]. In 2015, in a multicenter, randomized, open-label, blinded endpoint, parallel group study, no significant differences were found between the two groups for the onset of stroke and for the occurrence of adverse events [24]. In conclusion, even if the action of statins on the prevention of atherosclerotic carotid plaque is well known, the neuroprotective effect of this molecule is still debated (Table 1).

Minocycline is a tetracycline antibiotic with anti-inflammatory, anti-apoptotic, and antioxidant effects that promote neuroprotection. Preclinical studies point out the efficacy of the molecule in reducing the infarct size [25]. The administration of minocycline in combination with t-PA were found to reduce brain injury and also the risk of infarction [26]. Clinical studies confirmed the safety of the administration of minocycline alone or in combination with tPA, even if little is known about its efficacy [27] (Table 1).

Albumin has various antioxidant effects and improves microvascular blood flow in the ischemic regions [28]. The ALIAS pilot trial showed that prognosis after the administration of albumin in combination with tPA was three times better in a high-dose albumin group compared to a low-dose group [29]. However, the analysis of the combined data from part one and two of the ALIAS trials showed that treatment with intravenous albumin, at 3 months, was associated with increased rates of adverse events such as intracerebral hemorrhage (Table 1).

Citicoline is a drug with a high capacity to enter the blood–brain barrier and an excellent safety profile [30]. This molecule plays a neuroprotective role, promoting membrane stability, and inhibiting excitotoxicity, oxidative stress, and apoptosis [31]. In preclinical studies, citicoline increased SIRT1 protein levels with concomitant neuroprotection [32]. Unexpectedly, a large multicenter European RCT (ICTUS trial) on patients treated with citicoline for 6 weeks, within 24 h from acute stroke, was stopped prematurely because no differences pointed out between citicoline and placebo groups [33]. However, a meta-analysis of acute ischemic stroke showed that patients who received the highest dose of citicoline, within the first 24 h, not treated with tPA, showed improvements [34] (Table 1).

Pioglitazone is an oral drug that reduces insulin resistance in type II diabetes [35]. A phase III trial (NCT00091949) in 2015 studied the efficacy of pioglitazone in non-diabetic patients who suffered from ischemic stroke in secondary prevention. All the participants in the study had insulin resistance and the true efficacy of the molecule in non-diabetic patients was not detectable (Table 1).

NA-1 plays a neuroprotective role in protecting neurons from excitotoxicity induced by the activation of NMDA receptors [36]. A phase III RCT (ESCAPE-NA1) evaluated the neuroprotective action of NA-1 in patients undergoing endovascular thrombectomy. NA-1 did not show any beneficial effects in patients who had good outcomes after endovascular treatment when compared with the placebo group. However, the beneficial effect of NA-1 showed in patients who did not receive endovascular treatment, with better outcomes and smaller infarction [37] (Table 1).

Hypothermia in stroke animal models seems to reduce metabolic demand, preserving energy, and decreasing glutamate and ROS with anti-inflammatory and anti-apoptotic effects. In stroke patients, hypothermia is obtained by using catheters introduced in the inferior vena cava or by surface cooling. Preliminary clinical studies point out no beneficial outcomes in terms of mortality [38,39] (Table 1).

Table 1. Common neuroprotective treatments, their mechanisms of action, and main outcomes.

Neuroprotective Factors	Mechanisms	Preclinical Outcome	Clinical Outcome
Anti excitotoxicity Magnesium sulfate [5] NA-1	blocking NMDA receptors reducing glutamate release blocking calcium channel inhibiting NMDA receptors	Effective	No convincing evidence
Antioxidant Ebselen [9] Edaravone [11]	ROS scavengers	Effective but narrow therapeutic window/study quality issues	Not effective Increased adverse events
Haematopoietic growth factor G-CSF [16] EPO [20]	reducing excitotoxicity anti-inflammatory and anti-apoptotic effect increasing neurogenesis	Effective but methodological bias	Not effective Increased adverse events
Statins [24]	inhibiting HMGCoA reductase	Effective but study quality issue	Contrasting results
Antibiotics Minocycline [25]	anti-inflammatory and anti-apoptotic effects	Effective	Safe No data about effeicacy
Albumin [29]	Improving microvascular blood flow	Effective	Increase adverse events
Neurovascular repair Citicoline [33]	promoting membrane stability inhibiting excitotoxicity, oxidative stress and apoptosis	Effective	Contrasting results
Pioglitazone [35]	No clear mechanism	Effective	Not detectable efficacy in non diabetic patient
Non pharmacological Hypotermia [39]	reducing metabolic demand preserving energy decreasing glutamate and ROS anti-inflammatory and anti-apoptotic effect	Effective	Management difficulties Adverse events

2. The Failure of Neuroprotection: From Bench to Bedside

The identification of pathways underlying cell death during ischemic damage has enabled the development of new promising neuroprotective drugs. To date, the results are linked to a complex transposition from the bench to the bedside table. This difficulty has spread pessimism about the potential role of these drugs in clinical practice [40].

Among these translational difficulties, the time of administration is crucial. In preclinical studies, neuroprotective agents are applied immediately after the mechanical occlusion of the vessel [41]. This is an unlikely condition in humans, where the exact time of symptom onset is not always known and the administration of the drug is unlikely to take place in a short time. Therefore, the administration of the agent at a variable time from the ischemic event could explain the heterogeneous response presented by patients towards the same neuroprotector.

Another difference between animal and clinical studies could relate to the affected vessels. In animal models, the vessel is closed mechanically and later reperfused. There is a concern that the infused drug will reach the ischemic zone more quickly compared to stroke patients who continue to have vessel occlusion [41].

Finally, preclinical studies use healthy animals of similar ages (typically rodents with less than 3 months of age). Human patients vary widely in the age range and usually have a variable comorbidity pattern [42].

3. Future Perspectives

The main purpose of stroke therapy is to restore cerebral blood flow after ischemic insult; the secondary purpose is to modulate the factors that could aggravate this damage and, if possible, to repair it [43].

The first problem in stroke patients is that not all of them can be revascularized, and therefore neuroprotective agents cannot sufficiently reach salvageable tissue. Moreover, many different processes occur consequently and synergistically during ischemic cascade: excitotoxicity, oxidative and nitrosative stress, inflammation, and reperfusion processes [42].

Preclinical trials combining different neuroprotective drugs (e.g., a cocktail with anti-excitotoxicity + anti-inflammatory + antioxidant properties) with vascular reperfusion therapy could represent effective future prospects in this area of research [44,45].

Moreover, good collateral circulation (pial and leptomeningeal collaterals) may improve stroke tolerance, due to fast neurological symptom improvements after thrombolytic and thrombectomy therapies and a reduction in intracranial hemorrhage risks [46].

Several strategies that could improve collateral circulation have been investigated, but none have been applicable in clinical practice [42].

Another important aspect of restoring brain damage is to prevent the no-reflow phenomenon and hemorrhagic transformation. Drugs alone have not been shown to protect the brain–blood barrier damage caused by various mechanisms during ischemia–reperfusion injury in human hemorrhagic transformation [42].

4. Conclusions

In conclusion, the development of neuroprotective therapies in stroke patients is assuming an increasingly central role in preclinical studies and, therefore, in those of translational medicine. This is related to the fact that multitarget neuroprotectants could represent a highly promising tool for improving stroke care. Future research should take into account a comprehensive strategy including neuroprotectant cocktails, mechanisms of reperfusion, angiogenesis, collateral circulations, and the prevention of post-ischemia hemorrhages.

Author Contributions: Conceptualization, L.G., C.C. and R.R.; writing—original draft preparation, L.G, C.C. and R.R.; writing—review and editing, L.G., C.C. and R.R.; supervision, L.G., C.C. and R.R. All authors have read and agreed to the published version of the manuscript.

Funding: This research received no external funding.

Acknowledgments: The completion of this research project would not have been possible without the contributions and support of many colleagues. We are deeply grateful to all those who played a role in the success of this project. We would like to thank Paciaroni for his invaluable input and support. His insights and expertise were instrumental in shaping the direction of this project.

Conflicts of Interest: The authors declare no conflict of interest.

References

1. Ginsberg, M.D. Neuroprotection for ischemic stroke: Past, present and future. *Neuropharmacology* **2008**, *55*, 363–389. [CrossRef] [PubMed]
2. Lai, T.W.; Zhang, S.; Wang, Y.T. Excitotoxicity and stroke: Identifying novel targets for neuroprotection. *Prog. Neurobiol.* **2014**, *115*, 157–188. [CrossRef] [PubMed]
3. Zhang, J.H.; Badaut, J.; Tang, J.; Obenaus, A.; Hartman, R.; Pearce, W.J. The vascular neural network—A new paradigm in stroke pathophysiology. *Nat. Rev. Neurol.* **2012**, *8*, 711–716. [CrossRef] [PubMed]
4. Iadecola, C.; Anrather, J. The immunology of stroke: From mechanisms to translation. *Nat. Med.* **2011**, *17*, 796–808. [CrossRef]
5. Westermaier, T.; Stetter, C.; Kunze, E.; Willner, N.; Raslan, F.; Vince, G.H.; Ernestus, R.-I. Magnesium treatment for neuroprotection in ischemic diseases of the brain. *Exp. Transl. Stroke Med.* **2013**, *5*, 6. [CrossRef]
6. Amaro, S.; Chamorro, A. Translational Stroke Research of the Combination of Thrombolysis and Antioxidant Therapy. *Stroke* **2011**, *42*, 1495–1499. [CrossRef]
7. Imai, H.; Graham, D.I.; Masayasu, H.; Macrae, I.M. Antioxidant ebselen reduces oxidative damage in focal cerebral ischemia. *Free. Radic. Biol. Med.* **2002**, *34*, 56–63. [CrossRef]
8. Lapchak, P.A. A critical assessment of edaravone acute ischemic stroke efficacy trials: Is edaravone an effective neuroprotective therapy? *Expert Opin. Pharmacother.* **2010**, *11*, 1753–1763. [CrossRef]
9. Ogawa, A.; Yoshimoto, T.; Kikuchi, H.; Sano, K.; Saito, I.; Yamaguchi, T.; Yasuhara, H.; for the Ebselen Study Group. Ebselen in Acute Middle Cerebral Artery Occlusion: A Placebo-Controlled, Double-Blind Clinical Trial. *Cerebrovasc. Dis.* **1999**, *9*, 112–118. [CrossRef]
10. Van Der Worp, H.B.; Macleod, M.R.; Bath, P.M.; Bathula, R.; Christensen, H.; Colam, B.; Cordonnier, C.; Demotes-Mainard, J.; Durand-Zaleski, I.; Gluud, C.; et al. Therapeutic hypothermia for acute ischaemic stroke. Results of a European multicentre, randomised, phase III clinical trial. *Eur. Stroke J.* **2019**, *4*, 254–262. [CrossRef]
11. Feng, S.; Yang, Q.; Liu, M.; Li, W.; Yuan, W.; Zhang, S.; Wu, B.; Li, J. Edaravone for acute ischaemic stroke. *Cochrane Database Syst. Rev.* **2011**, CD007230. [CrossRef]
12. Kono, S.; Deguchi, K.; Morimoto, N.; Kurata, T.; Yamashita, T.; Ikeda, Y.; Narai, H.; Manabe, Y.; Takao, Y.; Kawada, S.; et al. Intraflen in Acute Middle Cerebral Artery Occlusion: A Placebo-Controlled, Double-Blinvenous Thrombolysis with Neuroprotective Therapy by Edaravone for Ischemic Stroke Patients Older than 80 Years of Age. *J. Stroke Cerebrovasc. Dis.* **2013**, *22*, 1175–1183. [CrossRef]

13. Minnerup, J.; Heidrich, J.; Wellmann, J.; Rogalewski, A.; Schneider, A.; Schäbitz, W.-R. Meta-Analysis of the Efficacy of Granulocyte-Colony Stimulating Factor in Animal Models of Focal Cerebral Ischemia. *Stroke* **2008**, *39*, 1855–1861. [CrossRef] [PubMed]
14. England, T.J.; Gibson, C.L.; Bath, P.M. Granulocyte-colony stimulating factor in experimental stroke and its effects on infarct size and functional outcome: A systematic review. *Brain Res. Rev.* **2009**, *62*, 71–82. [CrossRef] [PubMed]
15. Schneider, A.; Wysocki, R.; Pitzer, C.; Krüger, C.; Laage, R.; Schwab, S.; Bach, A.; Schäbitz, W.-R. An extended window of opportunity for G-CSF treatment in cerebral ischemia. *BMC Biol.* **2006**, *4*, 36. [CrossRef] [PubMed]
16. Ringelstein, E.B.; Thijs, V.; Norrving, B.; Chamorro, A.; Aichner, F.; Grond, M.; Saver, J.; Laage, R.; Schneider, A.; Rathgeb, F.; et al. Granulocyte Colony–Stimulating Factor in Patients with Acute Ischemic Stroke. *Stroke* **2013**, *44*, 2681–2687. [CrossRef]
17. Bath, P.M.W.; Sprigg, N.; England, T. Colony stimulating factors (including erythropoietin, granulocyte colony stimulating factor and analogues) for stroke. *Cochrane Database Syst. Rev.* **2013**, *6*, CD005207. [CrossRef] [PubMed]
18. Minnerup, J.; Heidrich, J.; Rogalewski, A.; Schäbitz, W.-R.; Wellmann, J. The Efficacy of Erythropoietin and Its Analogues in Animal Stroke Models. *Stroke* **2009**, *40*, 3113–3120. [CrossRef]
19. Jerndal, M.; Forsberg, K.; Sena, E.S.; Macleod, M.R.; O'Collins, V.E.; Linden, T.K.; Nilsson, M.; Howells, D.W. A Systematic Review and Meta-Analysis of Erythropoietin in Experimental Stroke. *J. Cereb. Blood Flow Metab.* **2009**, *30*, 961–968. [CrossRef]
20. Ehrenreich, H.; Weissenborn, K.; Prange, H.; Schneider, D.; Weimar, C.; Wartenberg, K.; Schellinger, P.D.; Bohn, M.; Becker, H.; Wegrzyn, M.; et al. Recombinant Human Erythropoietin in the Treatment of Acute Ischemic Stroke. *Stroke* **2009**, *40*, e647–e656. [CrossRef]
21. Goldstein, L.B. Statins and ischemic stroke severity: Cytoprotection. *Curr. Atheroscler. Rep.* **2009**, *11*, 296–300. [CrossRef] [PubMed]
22. Chróinín, D.N.; Asplund, K.; Åsberg, S.; Callaly, E.L.; Cuadrado-Godia, E.; Díez-Tejedor, E.; Di Napoli, M.; Engelter, S.T.; Furie, K.L.; Giannopoulos, S.; et al. Statin Therapy and Outcome After Ischemic Stroke. *Stroke* **2013**, *44*, 448–456. [CrossRef]
23. Cappellari, M.; Bovi, P.; Moretto, G.; Zini, A.; Nencini, P.; Sessa, M.; Furlan, M.; Pezzini, A.; Orlandi, G.; Paciaroni, M.; et al. The THRombolysis and STatins (THRaST) study. *Neurology* **2013**, *80*, 655–661. [CrossRef] [PubMed]
24. Hosomi, N.; Nagai, Y.; Kohriyama, T.; Ohtsuki, T.; Aoki, S.; Nezu, T.; Maruyama, H.; Sunami, N.; Yokota, C.; Kitagawa, K.; et al. The Japan Statin Treatment Against Recurrent Stroke (J-STARS): A Multicenter, Randomized, Open-label, Parallel-group Study. *Ebiomedicine* **2015**, *2*, 1071–1078. [CrossRef]
25. Liao, T.V.; Forehand, C.C.; Hess, D.C.; Fagan, S.C. Minocycline repurposing in critical illness: Focus on stroke. *Curr. Top. Med. Chem.* **2013**, *13*, 2283–2290. [CrossRef] [PubMed]
26. Fan, X.; Lo, E.H.; Wang, X. Effects of Minocycline Plus Tissue Plasminogen Activator Combination Therapy After Focal Embolic Stroke in Type 1 Diabetic Rats. *Stroke* **2013**, *44*, 745–752. [CrossRef] [PubMed]

27. Fagan, S.C.; Waller, J.L.; Nichols, F.T.; Edwards, D.J.; Pettigrew, L.C.; Clark, W.M.; Hall, C.E.; Switzer, J.A.; Ergul, A.; Hess, D.C.; et al. Minocycline to Improve Neurologic Outcome in Stroke (MINOS). *Stroke* **2010**, *41*, 2283–2287. [CrossRef]
28. Nimmagadda, A.; Park, H.-P.; Prado, R.; Ginsberg, M.D. Albumin Therapy Improves Local Vascular Dynamics in a Rat Model of Primary Microvascular Thrombosis. *Stroke* **2008**, *39*, 198–204. [CrossRef]
29. Palesch, Y.Y.; Hill, M.D.; Ryckborst, K.J.; Tamariz, D.; Ginsberg, M.D. The ALIAS Pilot Trial. *Stroke* **2006**, *37*, 2107–2114. [CrossRef]
30. Overgaard, K. The Effects of Citicoline on Acute Ischemic Stroke: A Review. *J. Stroke Cerebrovasc. Dis.* **2014**, *23*, 1764–1769. [CrossRef]
31. Wignall, N.D.; Brown, E.S. Citicoline in addictive disorders: A review of the literature. *Am. J. Drug Alcohol Abus.* **2014**, *40*, 262–268. [CrossRef] [PubMed]
32. Hurtado, O.; Hernández-Jiménez, M.; Zarruk, J.G.; Cuartero, M.I.; Ballesteros, I.; Camarero, G.; Moraga, A.; Pradillo, J.M.; Moro, M.A.; Lizasoain, I. Citicoline (CDP-choline) increases Sirtuin1 expression concomitant to neuroprotection in experimental stroke. *J. Neurochem.* **2013**, *126*, 819–826. [CrossRef] [PubMed]
33. Dávalos, A.; Alvarez-Sabín, J.; Castillo, J.; Díez-Tejedor, E.; Ferro, J.; Martínez-Vila, E.; Serena, J.; Segura, T.; Cruz, V.T.; Masjuan, J.; et al. Citicoline in the treatment of acute ischaemic stroke: An international, randomised, multicentre, placebo-controlled study (ICTUS trial). *Lancet* **2012**, *380*, 349–357. [CrossRef] [PubMed]
34. Secades, J.J.; Alvarez-Sabín, J.; Castillo, J.; Díez-Tejedor, E.; Martínez-Vila, E.; Ríos, J.; Oudovenko, N. Citicoline for Acute Ischemic Stroke: A Systematic Review and Formal Meta-analysis of Randomized, Double-Blind, and Placebo-Controlled Trials. *J. Stroke Cerebrovasc. Dis.* **2016**, *25*, 1984–1996. [CrossRef]
35. Yu, S.-J.; Reiner, D.; Shen, H.; Wu, K.-J.; Liu, Q.-R.; Wang, Y. Time-Dependent Protection of CB2 Receptor Agonist in Stroke. *PLoS ONE* **2015**, *10*, e0132487. [CrossRef] [PubMed]
36. Ballarin, B.; Tymianski, M. Discovery and development of NA-1 for the treatment of acute ischemic stroke. *Acta Pharmacol. Sin.* **2018**, *39*, 661–668. [CrossRef]
37. Hill, M.D.; Goyal, M.; Menon, B.K.; Nogueira, R.G.; A McTaggart, R.; Demchuk, A.M.; Poppe, A.Y.; Buck, B.H.; Field, T.S.; Dowlatshahi, D.; et al. Efficacy and safety of nerinetide for the treatment of acute ischaemic stroke (ESCAPE-NA1): A multicentre, double-blind, randomised controlled trial. *Lancet* **2020**, *395*, 878–887. [CrossRef]
38. Lakhan, S.E.; Pamplona, F. Application of Mild Therapeutic Hypothermia on Stroke: A Systematic Review and Meta-Analysis. *Stroke Res. Treat.* **2012**, *2012*, 295906. [CrossRef]
39. Hertog, H.M.D.; Van Der Worp, H.B.; Tseng, M.-C.; Dippel, D.W. Cooling therapy for acute stroke. *Cochrane Database Syst. Rev.* **2009**, *2009*, CD001247. [CrossRef]
40. Minnerup, J.; Sutherland, B.A.; Buchan, A.M.; Kleinschnitz, C. Neuroprotection for Stroke: Current Status and Future Perspectives. *Int. J. Mol. Sci.* **2012**, *13*, 11753–11772. [CrossRef]
41. Grupke, S.; Hall, J.; Dobbs, M.; Bix, G.J.; Fraser, J.F. Understanding history, and not repeating it. Neuroprotection for acute ischemic stroke: From review to preview. *Clin. Neurol. Neurosurg.* **2015**, *129*, 1–9. [CrossRef]
42. Xiong, X.-Y.; Liu, L.; Yang, Q.-W. Refocusing Neuroprotection in Cerebral Reperfusion Era: New Challenges and Strategies. *Front. Neurol.* **2018**, *9*, 249. [CrossRef] [PubMed]

43. Neuhaus, A.; Couch, Y.; Hadley, G.; Buchan, A.M. Neuroprotection in stroke: The importance of collaboration and reproducibility. *Brain* **2017**, *140*, 2079–2092. [CrossRef] [PubMed]
44. Xiong, X.-Y.; Liu, L.; Yang, Q.-W. Functions and mechanisms of microglia/macrophages in neuroinflammation and neurogenesis after stroke. *Prog. Neurobiol.* **2016**, *142*, 23–44. [CrossRef] [PubMed]
45. Garber, K. Stroke treatment—Light at the end of the tunnel? *Nat. Biotechnol.* **2007**, *25*, 838–840. [CrossRef]
46. Leng, X.; Lan, L.; Liu, L.; Leung, T.W.; Wong, K.S. Good collateral circulation predicts favorable outcomes in intravenous thrombolysis: A systematic review and meta-analysis. *Eur. J. Neurol.* **2016**, *23*, 1738–1749. [CrossRef]

© 2023 by the authors. Licensee MDPI, Basel, Switzerland. This article is an open access article distributed under the terms and conditions of the Creative Commons Attribution (CC BY) license (http://creativecommons.org/licenses/by/4.0/).

Stroke Rehabilitation from a Historical Perspective

Monica Acciarresi and Mauro Zampolini

Abstract: In western industrialized countries, stroke is one of the leading causes of acquired adult disability. Because of the recent advances in acute stroke treatment and neurocritical care, more patients survive stroke, with varying degrees of disability. Stroke rehabilitation is a dynamically changing field that is increasingly expanding. Advances in knowledge of mechanisms underlying stroke recovering and in technology are aiding the development of therapies that requires a multidisciplinary approach by physicians, therapists, biologists, physiologist and engineers working together with the aim of improve the quality of life of patients with stroke.

1. Introduction

Stroke is highly associated with acquired disability in developed nations [1]. Progress of late, in both acute stroke and neurocritical care, has led to greater numbers of stroke survivors; however, too often, survivors are burdened with acquired stroke disability [2].

It is widely known that observed neurological deficits are important for indicating the locations of damage done to tissue, as well as any associated neuronal loss [3], which, in turn, is responsible for the burden of disability [4].

2. Stroke Recovery and Stroke Rehabilitation

Generally speaking, stroke rehabilitation is commonly defined as any form of stroke care that seeks to reduce disability, while at the same time, foster more active participation in daily living activities. Achieving the highest possible level of independence is of paramount importance [2].

Stroke recovery focuses on striving to increase performance- and activity-based behavioral targets [2]. Recovery is recognized as being an articulated process, which can be successfully achieved when a combination of spontaneous and learning-dependent processes are improved upon. These include restitution, substitution and compensation. By definition, the first of these strives to regain functionality of any impaired neural tissue; the second reorganizes untouched neural pathways, so to regain functioning; whilst the third seeks to obtain betterment with regard to the issue of disparity between the impaired skills [5]. Despite the fact that patient outcome tends to be heterogeneous and individual recoveries differ widely due to varying patient features, results from several cohort studies [6] have reported that recovery can be predicted for the first few days post-event.

The ability to more accurately predict recovery on an individual level has been enhanced through the development of a multimodal biomarker-based algorithm based upon clinical results, for the most part made up of neurophysiological and brain imaging results [7]. Specifically, if patients exhibit the marked impairment of both shoulder abduction and finger extension, the functional integrity of the corticospinal tract can be assessed using transcranial magnetic brain stimulation. Whenever a motor-evoked potential is recorded, a good recovery can be predicted, as the tract will still be intact [8].

Currently, international guidelines recommend that any stroke rehabilitation regimen be performed under the direction of a qualified Stroke Unit, incorporating multidisciplinary rehabilitation strategies, within a few days of an event [9,10]. To this regard, the literature published to date suggests that intensive rehabilitation, when led by a structured multidisciplinary team, will more likely produce greater benefits, in terms of outcome and/or alleviating the burden of disability; in fact, results reported by less intense programs without the direction of a multidisciplinary team have failed to match these levels of benefit [11].

With regard to behavioral recovery, on average, it will occur within the first three months after stroke. In animal models, researchers have reported that any postponement in training after stroke, in animal models, was associated with attenuated effectiveness. However, results from clinical studies on this topic have not been so straightforward [12]. In fact, findings from human trials suggest that rehabilitation might be harmful when hastily initiated. The AVERT trial findings suggest that immediate mobilization, on average $\approx$ 18 h after stroke, was associated with a reduction in favorable outcome at 90 days [13].

To date, no moderate nonlinear association between impairment and function has been reported, particularly for motor impairment [5,6,14]. Moreover, evidence of neurological repair associated with the use of impairment-focused therapies has yet to be demonstrated. On the other hand, strong evidence exists supporting the role of task-oriented training. Here, the focus is on bolstering the natural pattern of functional recovery, driven mainly by adaptive strategies that make up for any impaired body functions [5,14,15].

Prior to current neurophysiological rehabilitation approaches, central nervous system damage had been treated via compensatory and orthopedic approaches: the stretching, bracing and strengthening of the affected side and by instructing patients to favor their sides unaffected by stroke [16]. A clearer understanding has been ascertained of the underlying mechanisms responsible for motor learning [17] and functional recovery post-stroke [5]. It seems that varying mechanisms trigger the nonlinear pattern of neurological recovery. To this regard, we mean the salvation of penumbral tissue surrounding the infarcted area; an elevation of cerebral shock, otherwise known as elevation of diaschisis; and finally, the ability of the brain to adapt via neuroplasticity [18].

Neuroplasticity, defined as changes in or a rewiring of the neural network, is held to be the main recovery process. The neural basis for post-stroke recovery relies on plasticity [19], namely, the ability of central nervous system cells to modify their structures and functioning in response to external stimuli [3]. Immediately following stroke, activation is decreased in the cortical areas afflicted, therein triggering changes in the localizations of certain tasks, such as movement.

During the acute and subacute phases, the neural networks will reconnect in the adjacent areas of the event site. However, in order to foster effective plasticity, rehabilitation interventions need to be task specific [2]. Recently developed neurorehabilitative approaches aim at stimulating cerebral plasticity through the employment of task-oriented models of motor learning [3,20–23].

3. New Neurorehabilitative Approches

Constraint-Induced Movement Therapy (CIMT) is a motor rehabilitation therapy technique that employs a mitt to constrain the unaffected limb, thereby the patient will favor the use of his/her affected hand. Clearly, the objective is to challenge the maladaptive "learned nonuse" of the paretic limb. This is achieved by not utilizing the compromised limb. Investigations made up of RCTs, along with a Cochrane review, have reported that CIMT played a role in augmenting the performance of motor skills [24,25], particularly with regard to arm function. It must be remembered that the routine use of CIMT is not without limitations. First of all, it is recognized as being labor-intensive, as well as being recommendable solely in those patients possessing discernable levels of conservation for motor skills performance. Moreover, any such candidates are required to have control over the functioning of their wrists and fingers.

Likewise, mirror therapy is an ulterior approach based on multisensory stimulation. This technique entails placing a mirror at a 90° angle in the midsagittal plane of the patient, so as to hide the paretic limb anterior to the mirror. Here, the unaffected limb is viewed, as if it were the affected arm, therein leading to the false perception on the part of the patient that the compromised limb is working regularly. Mirror therapy effects may influence the activity of mirror neurons [26]. A review [27] including 14 studies including 567 enrolled subjects who had utilized mirror therapy reported that, compared to other approaches, the former was associated with a greater impact with regard to benefiting motor function.

Virtual reality technologies are novel rehabilitation approaches utilizing interaction with virtual elements found in the environment [28]. A Cochrane review [29] reported a paucity of proof regarding the hypothesis claiming that virtual reality and interactive exercises might be associated with a greater benefit in daily functioning, compared to conventional treatments. Results from a meta-analysis on virtual reality [30] found that most of the included studies had reported evidence of significant motor recoveries after stroke for the upper limbs. Data from randomized controlled trials are needed to confirm this finding.

Robot-assisted rehabilitative devices have been shown to facilitate upper limb motor recovery in the absence of a significant benefit with regard to functional ability [31]. Specifically, in the UL-Robot Trial [32], one group received robot-assisted therapy, and the second group was prescribed standard physical therapy. The two groups were each compared to a cohort prescribed standard care. Whilst a superiority of the former therapy over the latter was not observed, both therapies did, however, prove to be better than standard care. Here, the authors suggested that the intensity of training might have acted decisively on motor recovery. Likewise, the Locomotor Experience Applied Post-Stroke (LEAPS) Trial, carried out by Duncan et al. [33], compared the impacts of robot-assisted rehabilitative devices through the employment of a body-weight-supported treadmill versus a standard home physical therapy program. The authors reported that most of the subjects (52%) referred to having improved walking function. However, no significant intergroup differences were recorded.

Concerning novel rehabilitation modalities, noninvasive brain stimulation techniques aimed at stimulating adaptative plasticity have produced beneficial early-phase results [34]. The theoretical model for brain stimulation is regarded as an "interhemispheric interaction" between the two primary motor cortices [35]. In healthy subjects, these cortices exert mutual inhibition at rest [8]. The interhemispheric competition model assumes that the unopposed excessive inhibition on the part of the healthy to the compromised hemisphere might hamper post stroke recovery. This theoretical model comprises (a) a post stroke imbalance of interhemispheric motor interactions, (b) diminished motor activity in the lesioned hemisphere and (c) overactive motor activity in the contralesional hemisphere.

The modulation of such an imbalance might foster motor recovery via brain stimulation in stroke survivors [34]. Presently, the two techniques for enabling enhancement and inhibition of a cortical nature [3] are repetitive transcranial magnetic stimulation (rTMS) and transcranial direct current stimulation (tDCS). In the former, a coil generates a focal magnetic field on the scalp, therein inducing, transiently, focally and reversibly, an electric current in the cortex below. Stimulation in the range of 1Hz alleviates cortical excitability, whereas greater frequencies raise cortical excitability. As for tDCS, weak direct currents are delivered to the cortex by way of two electrodes that aim to polarize the underlying tissue.

Correct electrode placement is required, so as to appropriately modulate both the current flow's distribution and direction. To this regard, anodal stimulation is associated with an excitatory effect through cortical neuron depolarization, whilst cathodal tDCS hyperpolarizes neurons via the suppression of cortical excitability.

Corti et al. [36] have suggested that rTMS is safe to use and could also be effective in facilitating motor recovery. Double-blinded, sham-controlled Phase II and Phase III clinical trials with larger sample sizes are needed to confirm this benefit. Hsu et al. performed a meta-analysis of 18 randomized controlled trials investigating rTMS benefit on upper limb motor impairment [37]. The authors, for motor outcome function, reported an associated benefit for subcortical stroke when low-frequency rTMS was applied to the unaffected hemisphere. Future well-designed randomized controlled trials are needed to confirm this finding. Results from a pilot randomized controlled trial performed by Kedhr et al. [38] showed that anodal and cathodal tDCS outperformed the sham stimulation with regard to the effects of rehabilitation of a training nature.

A review [34] of published tDCS studies reported positive stroke recovery results. However, albeit a large multicenter randomized study, most of the included studies were proof-of-concept investigations having limited sample sizes [35]. The current issues in current tDCS research for stroke recovery include the determination of optimal dosages and montages, the obtainment of reliable data able to predict long-term safety profiles, and finally, how to achieve a better estimate of the effect size of tDCS.

4. Conclusions

Stroke rehabilitation is a continuously evolving field. A greater understanding of the mechanisms underlying stroke recovery, along with advances in technology, are allowing for the development of more effective approaches able to effectively alleviate the burden of acquired stroke disability. In addition, when led by a structured multidisciplinary team, these regimens will more likely determine greater benefits.

Author Contributions: M.A. has drafted the work and M.Z. substantively revised it. Both the authors have approved the submitted version and agrees to be personally accountable for the author's own contributions and for ensuring that questions related to the accuracy or integrity of any part of the work, even ones in which the author was not personally involved, are appropriately investigated, resolved, and documented in the literature. All authors have read and agreed to the published version of the manuscript.

Funding: This research received no external funding.

Acknowledgments: The authors thank Paciaroni for the invitation to participate in this publication.

Conflicts of Interest: The authors declare no conflict of interest.

References

1. Kolominsky-Rabas, P.L.; Weber, M.; Gefeller, O.; Neundoerfer, B.; Heuschmann, P.U. Epidemiology of ischemic stroke subtypes according to TOAST criteria: Incidence, recurrence, and long-term survival in ischemic stroke subtypes: A population-based study. *Stroke* **2001**, *1*, 2735–2740. [CrossRef]
2. Belagaje, S.R. Stroke Rehabilitation. *Continuum (Minneap Minn)* **2017**, *23*, 238–253. [CrossRef]
3. Faralli, A.; Bigoni, M.; Mauro, A.; Rossi, F.; Carulli, D. Noninvasive strategies to promote functional recovery after stroke. *Neural Plast.* **2013**, *2013*, 854597. [CrossRef]
4. WHO. The World Health Report 2003: Shaping the Future. October 2003. Available online: http://www.who.int/whr/2003/en/overview_en.pdf (accessed on 7 September 2010).
5. Kwakkel, G.; Kollen, B.; Lindeman, E. Understanding the pattern of functional recovery after stroke: Facts and theories. *Restor. Neurol. Neurosci.* **2004**, *22*, 281–299.

6. Nijland, R.; van Wegen, E.E.; Verbunt, J.; van Wijk, R.; van Kordelaar, J.; Kwakkel, G. A comparison of two validated tests for upper limb function after stroke: The Wolf Motor Function Test and the Action Research Arm Test. *J. Rehabil. Med.* **2010**, *42*, 694–696.
7. Roemmich, R.T.; Bastian, A.J. Closing the loop: From motor neuroscience to neurorehabilitation. *Annu. Rev. Neurosci.* **2018**, *41*, 415–429. [CrossRef]
8. Anaya, A.M.; Branscheidt, M. Neurorehabilitation after stroke: From bedside to the laboratory and back. *Stroke* **2019**, *50*, e180–e182. [CrossRef]
9. Bernhardt, J.; Thuy, N.; Collier, J.M.; Legg, L.A. Very early versus delayed mobilisation after stroke. *Cochrane Database Syst. Rev.* **2009**, *1*, IDCD006187. [CrossRef]
10. Stroke Unit Trialists' Collaboration. Organised inpatient (stroke unit) care for stroke. *Cochrane Database Syst. Rev.* **2002**, *1*, CD000197.
11. The European Stroke Organisation (ESO) Executive Committee and the ESO Writing Committee. Guidelines for management of ischaemic stroke and transient ischaemic attack. *Cerebrovasc. Dis.* **2008**, *25*, 457–507. [CrossRef]
12. Coleman, E.R.; Moudgal, R.; Lang, K.; Hyacinth, H.I.; Awosika, O.O.; Kissela, B.M.; Feng, W. Early rehabilitation after stroke: A narrative review. *Curr. Atheroscler. Rep.* **2017**, *19*, 59. [CrossRef] [PubMed]
13. Lang, C.E.; Strube, M.J.; Bland, M.D.; Waddell, K.J.; Cherry-Allen, K.M.; Nudo, R.J.; Dromerick, A.W.; Birkenmeier, R.L. Dose response of task-specific upper limb training in people at least 6 months poststroke: A phase II, single-blind, randomized, controlled trial. *Ann. Neurol.* **2016**, *80*, 342–354. [CrossRef]
14. Levin, M.F.; Kleim, J.A.; Wolf, S.L. What do motor "recovery" and "compensation" mean in patients following stroke? *Neurorehabil. Neural Repair* **2009**, *23*, 313–319. [CrossRef]
15. Murphy, T.H.; Corbett, D. Plasticity during stroke recovery: From synapse to behaviour. *Nat. Rev. Neurosci.* **2009**, *10*, 861–872. [CrossRef]
16. Lennon, S. The Bobath Concept: A critical review of the theoretical assumptions that guide physiotherapy practice in stroke rehabilitation. *Phys. Ther. Rev.* **1996**, *1*, 35–45. [CrossRef]
17. Dobkin, B.H. Presence of finger extension and shoulder abduction within 72 h after stroke predicts functional recovery: Early prediction of functional outcome after stroke: The EPOS cohort study. *Neurorehabil. Neural Repair* **2007**, *21*, 3–13. [CrossRef]
18. Kollen, B.J.; Lennon, S.; Lyons, B.; Wheatley-Smith, L.; Scheper, M.; Buurke, J.H.; Halfens, J.; Geurts, A.C.; Kwakkel, G. The effectiveness of the Bobath concept in stroke rehabilitation: What is the evidence? *Stroke* **2009**, *40*, e89–e97. [CrossRef]
19. Carmichael, S.T. Targets for neural repair therapies after stroke. *Stroke* **2010**, *41*, 124–126. [CrossRef] [PubMed]
20. Kwakkel, G.; Wagenaar, R.C.; Twisk, J.W.; Lankhorst, G.J.; Koetsier, J.C. Intensity of leg and arm training after primary middle-cerebral-artery stroke: A randomised trial. *Lancet* **1999**, *354*, 191–196. [CrossRef] [PubMed]
21. Macko, R.F.; Ivey, F.M.; Forrester, L.W. Task-oriented aerobic exercise in chronic hemiparetic stroke: Training protocols and treatment effects. *Top. Stroke Rehabil.* **2005**, *12*, 45–57. [CrossRef]

22. Van De Port, I.G.; Wood-Dauphinee, S.; Lindeman, E.; Kwakkel, G. Effects of exercise training programs on walking competency after stroke: A systematic review. *Am. J. Phys. Med. Rehabil.* **2007**, *86*, 935–951. [CrossRef] [PubMed]
23. Govender, P.; Kalra, L. Benefits of occupational therapy in stroke rehabilitation. *Expert Rev. Neurother.* **2007**, *7*, 1013–1019. [CrossRef] [PubMed]
24. Wolf, S.L.; Winstein, C.J.; Miller, J.P.; Taub, E.; Uswatte, G.; Morris, D.; Giuliani, C.; Light, K.E.; Nichols-Larsen, D.; for the EXCITE Investigators. Effect of constraintinduced movement therapy on upper extremity function 3 to 9 months after stroke: The EXCITE randomized clinical trial. *JAMA* **2006**, *296*, 2095–2104. [CrossRef] [PubMed]
25. Sirtori, V.; Corbetta, D.; Moja, L.; Gatti, R. Constraintinduced movement therapy for upper extremities in stroke patients. *Cochrane Database Syst. Rev.* **2009**, *4*, CD004433.
26. Rizzolatti, G.; Sinigaglia, C. The functional role of the parieto-frontal mirror circuit: Interpretations and misinterpretations. *Nat. Rev. Neurosci.* **2010**, *11*, 264–274. [CrossRef] [PubMed]
27. Thieme, H.; Mehrholz, J.; Pohl, M.; Behrens, J.; Dohle, C. Mirror therapy for improving motor function after stroke. *Cochrane Database Syst. Rev.* 2012 3, CD008449.
28. Sveistrup, H. Motor rehabilitation using virtual reality. *J. NeuroEng. Rehabil.* **2004**, *1*, 10. [CrossRef]
29. Laver, K.E.; Lange, B.; George, S.; Deutsch, J.E.; Saposnik, G.; Crotty, M. Virtual reality for stroke rehabilitation. *Cochrane Database Syst. Rev.* **2011**, *11*, CD008349.
30. Saposnik, G.; Levin, M. Virtual reality in stroke rehabilitation: A meta-analysis and implications for clinicians. *Stroke* **2011**, *42*, 1380–1386. [CrossRef] [PubMed]
31. Kwakkel, G.; Kollen, B.J.; Krebs, H.I. Effects of robotassisted therapy on upper limb recovery after stroke: A systematic review. *Neurorehabilit. Neural Repair* **2008**, *22*, 111–121. [CrossRef]
32. Lo, A.C.; Guarino, P.D.; Richards, L.G.; Haselkorn, J.K.; Wittenberg, G.F.; Federman, D.G.; Ringer, R.J.; Wagner, T.H.; Krebs, H.I.; Volpe, B.T.; et al. Robot-assisted therapy for long-termupper-limb impairment after stroke. *N. Engl. J. Med.* **2010**, *362*, 1772–1783. [CrossRef]
33. Duncan, P.W.; Sullivan, K.J.; Behrman, A.L.; Azen, S.P.; Wu, S.S.; Nadeau, S.E.; Dobkin, B.H.; Rose, D.K.; Tilson, J.K.; Cen, S.; et al. Body-weight-supported treadmill rehabilitation after stroke. *N. Engl. J. Med.* **2011**, *364*, 2026–2036. [CrossRef]
34. Feng, W.W.; Bowden, M.G.; Kautz, S. Review of transcranial direct current stimulation in poststroke recovery. *Top. Stroke Rehabil.* **2013**, *20*, 68–77. [CrossRef]
35. Perez, M.A.; Cohen, L.G. Interhemispheric inhibition between primary motor cortices: What have we learned? *J. Physiol.* **2009**, *587*, 725–726. [CrossRef]
36. Corti, M.; Patten, C.; Triggs, W. Repetitive transcranial magnetic stimulation of motor cortex after stroke: A focused review. *Am. J. Phys. Med. Rehabil.* **2012**, *91*, 254–270. [CrossRef]
37. Hsu, W.Y.; Cheng, C.H.; Liao, K.K.; Lee, I.H.; Lin, Y.Y. Effects of repetitive transcranial magnetic stimulation on motor functions in patients with stroke: A meta-analysis. *Stroke* **2012**, *43*, 1849–1857. [CrossRef]

38. Khedr, E.M.; Shawky, O.A.; El-Hammady, D.H.; Rothwell, J.C.; Darwish, E.S.; Mostafa, O.M.; Tohamy, A.M. Effect of anodal versus cathodal transcranial direct current stimulation on stroke rehabilitation: A pilot randomized controlled trial. *Neurorehabilit. Neural Repair* **2013**, *27*, 592–601. [CrossRef]

© 2023 by the authors. Licensee MDPI, Basel, Switzerland. This article is an open access article distributed under the terms and conditions of the Creative Commons Attribution (CC BY) license (http://creativecommons.org/licenses/by/4.0/).

MDPI
St. Alban-Anlage 66
4052 Basel
Switzerland
www.mdpi.com

MDPI Books Editorial Office
E-mail: books@mdpi.com
www.mdpi.com/books

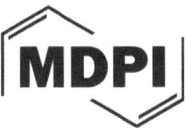

Disclaimer/Publisher's Note: The statements, opinions and data contained in all publications are solely those of the individual author(s) and contributor(s) and not of MDPI and/or the editor(s). MDPI and/or the editor(s) disclaim responsibility for any injury to people or property resulting from any ideas, methods, instructions or products referred to in the content.

www.ingramcontent.com/pod-product-compliance
Lightning Source LLC
LaVergne TN
LVHW072311090526
838202LV00018B/2261